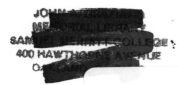

7/16/98

Understanding

Magnetic Resonance Imaging

Robert C. Smith
and
Robert C. Lange

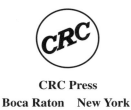

CRC Press
Boca Raton   New York

Acquiring Editor:	Marsha Baker
Project Editor:	Albert W. Starkweather, Jr.
Cover design:	Dawn Boyd

Library of Congress Cataloging-in-Publication Data

Smith, Robert C. (Robert Carl), 1960–
    Understanding magnetic resonance imaging / Robert C. Smith and Robert C. Lange.
       p. cm.
    Includes bibliographical references and index.
    ISBN 0-8493-2658-3 (alk. paper)
    1. Magnetic Resonance Imaging.I. Lange, Robert C.II. Title.
QC762.6.M34S65   1997
538′.362—dc21

                       97-29079
                        CIP

Dedications

For BJ

Robert C. Lange

To my family, for their enthusiastic encouragement and support.
To the Yale Radiology residents and fellows,
whose interest in understanding the technical aspects
of MRI prompted the work on this book.

Robert C. Smith

The Authors

Robert C. Lange was born and raised in the Boston area. He received a B.S. in Chemistry at Northeastern University in 1957, and a Ph.D. in Inorganic and Nuclear Chemistry at the Massachusetts Institute of Technology in 1962. After seven years of low-energy nuclear physics research at Mound Laboratory, Miamisburg, Ohio, he came to Yale University School of Medicine as a physicist in the Nuclear Medicine Section of the Department of Radiology. In 1986, he joined the Magnetic Resonance Imaging Section when MRI was introduced at the Yale–New Haven Medical Center. He is certified in Diagnostic Radiology and Nuclear Medicine Physics by the American Board of Radiology. His interests in MRI extend to safety and efficacy studies, and the evaluation of new hardware and software technology. He is the primary physics instructor for Diagnostic Radiology residents at Yale, teaching Diagnostic Radiology and Magnetic Resonance Imaging Physics.

Robert C. Smith was born in Brooklyn, New York in 1960. He was educated in the New York City public school system through high school. Dr. Smith received his B.A. degree in mathematics from The Johns Hopkins University in 1981 and his M.D. degree from Yale University in 1985. After completing his residency training in Diagnostic Radiology at Yale, Dr. Smith completed a fellowship in Magnetic Resonance Imaging. His interests in MRI include all technical aspects of imaging, pulse sequence development and testing, as well as all clinical applications of MRI to body imaging. He is currently Associate Professor at the Yale University School of Medicine and has served as Director of the Abdominal Imaging Fellowship Program as well as Chief of Magnetic Resonance Imaging.

Acknowledgments

To Janet W, Debbie M, and Kari K for their support and assistance during the construction of the book figures.

Preface

Magnetic resonance imaging (MRI) is based on the phenomenon of nuclear magnetic resonance (NMR). Although *nuclear* (N) has been dropped from the name, the phenomenon does originate in the nuclei of atoms. In order to perform and interpret MRI studies, an understanding of the basic underlying physical principles is essential. This book is intended for those readers with an interest in understanding the physical basis of MRI. Topics are discussed in a qualitative manner whenever possible. The number of mathematical equations is kept to a minimum. When equations are required, a qualitative explanation is also given and the complexity of the mathematics is usually kept at a low level.

The first four chapters review the basics of electricity and magnetism as well as the design and components of an MR imaging system. Chapters 5 and 6 discuss the interaction of the main magnetic field as well as the magnetic field of the external RF radiation with protons to produce an MR signal. The molecular basis and a detailed discussion of the meanings of T1 and T2 relaxation are given. Chapter 7 provides an overview of the entire imaging process including a detailed discussion of spin echo pulse sequences. Chapter 8 describes the Fourier transform process in order to provide an in-depth understanding of both phase and frequency encoding as well as precisely how the MR signal is measured. Chapter 9 provides a simple discussion of how different MR pulse sequence parameters affect the signal-to-noise ratio of an MR image.

Chapter 10 gives a comprehensive review of all currently utilized imaging options and methods to reduce image artifacts. This includes a detailed discussion of precisely how each option works and when it should be used. Chapter 11 describes all commonly used pulse sequences (other than conventional spin echo) with particular attention to gradient echo and fast spin echo sequences. The discussion of gradient echo sequences takes a generic approach and describes the underlying basis principles rather than the myriad of acronyms used to characterize these sequences. The origin of stimulated echoes is also provided in detail. The discussion of fast spin echo pulse sequences draws on the description of the Fourier transform process of Chapter 8 in order to explain the different contrast characteristics and imaging options of this important pulse sequence. Chapter 12 provides a brief description of multicoil technology and design. Chapter 13 reviews in detail both time-of-flight and phase contrast MR angiography. Finally, Chapter 14 discusses the origin and appearance of all of the commonly encountered MR image artifacts.

Table of Contents

1 Atoms and Nuclei

All matter within the universe consists of atoms, which are made up of protons, neutrons, and electrons. These three elementary particles are easily described by their physical properties:

Particle	Mass	Charge
Electron	9×10^{-30} kg	One negative charge
Proton	1.8×10^{-27} kg	One positive charge
Neutron	1.8×10^{-27} kg	Uncharged (neutral)

Protons and neutrons (collectively referred to as nucleons) are located in the nuclei of atoms, while the electrons are constrained to revolve around the nucleus in discrete shells (or orbits). The nucleus is the central, heavy, positively charged part of an atom and makes up most of the atom's mass. The nucleus is exceedingly small and dense (with a density of about 10^{15} g/cm^3). The nuclear radius is on the order of 10^{-15} m, compared with the atomic radius of about 10^{-10} m.

Atoms are characterized as a particular element by the number of protons within the nucleus, called the atomic number (Z). On the earth, atoms with atomic numbers between 1 and 92 occur naturally, but technetium (Tc, Z = 43) and promethium (Pm, Z = 61) are missing. These elements are radioactive and have short half-lives compared to the age of the earth. The number of neutrons in the nucleus of an atom is called the neutron number (N). In nature, stable (not radioactive) nuclei have $N \geq Z$. The nucleus of a given element can contain different numbers of neutrons (these are referred to as isotopes). On the earth, atoms with N between 0 and 146 can be found. The sum (N + Z) for an atom is called the mass number (A). An isotope of a given element (E) is usually denoted $^A_Z E_N$.

Nucleons in the nucleus are held together by the nuclear "strong" force — an attractive force that operates only at very short distances (about the nuclear radius). In addition, both protons and neutrons like to be paired (i.e., this is a more stable configuration). Nuclei with an even Z and an even N are much more stable than those with an odd Z and/or an odd N, as indicated in the following table:

Z	N	A	# Stable Isotopes	NMR Active
Even	Even	Even	165	No
Even	Odd	Odd	55	Yes
Odd	Even	Odd	50	Yes
Odd	Odd	Even	4	Yes

The last column shows that only those atoms with an odd number of protons (Z) or an odd number of neutrons (N) or with both odd, are NMR active. With regard to NMR activity, a number of biologically important atoms fortunately fall in the active category:

Z	N	Element	Isotope	% Abundance	Nuclear Spin
1	0	Hydrogen	^{1}H	99.98	1/2
1	1	Hydrogen	^{2}H	0.02	1
6	7	Carbon	^{13}C	1.10	1/2
7	7	Nitrogen	^{14}N	99.62	1
7	8	Nitrogen	^{15}N	0.38	1/2
8	9	Oxygen	^{17}O	0.039	5/2
9	10	Fluorine	^{19}F	100.0	1/2
11	12	Sodium	^{23}Na	100.0	3/2
12	13	Magnesium	^{25}Mg	11.50	5/2
15	16	Phosphorus	^{31}P	100.0	1/2
17	18	Chlorine	^{35}Cl	75.40	3/2
17	20	Chlorine	^{37}Cl	24.60	3/2
19	20	Potassium	^{39}K	93.38	3/2

The reason that these nuclei are NMR active derives from the property of nuclear spin. Nuclear spin (or just spin) results in elementary particles and some nuclei (which contain elementary particles) having associated with them an intrinsic magnetic field. For most of this discussion, the emphasis will be on the nucleus of the more abundant stable isotope of hydrogen, ^{1}H, which consists of a single proton. Explanations of physical phenomena will concentrate on the proton or a collection of protons in hydrogen-containing molecules such a water or lipids.

Moving charged particles give rise to a magnetic field. The simplest example is a current-carrying wire. When electric current runs through a wire, it is carried by electrons. If a magnetic material is placed near the current-carrying wire, it will experience a force that is dependent upon the magnitude and direction of the current in the wire as well as the distance from the wire. This force is described by the magnetic field associated with the current-carrying wire. Unlike the gravitational force, the magnetic force can be attractive or repulsive.

Independent of the magnetic field associated with their movement through space, elementary particles also possess an intrinsic magnetic field due to nuclear spin. Spin is an intrinsic angular momentum (i.e., rotational type motion) that can be crudely thought of as the particle spinning about its own axis. This spinning motion of a charged particle (e.g., an electron or proton) or even a neutral particle with an uneven charge distribution (e.g., a neutron) gives rise to a magnetic field. Experiments have demonstrated that nuclei with odd A or odd Z and odd N possess a net spin.

Like all atomic and nuclear properties, nuclear spin is quantized; that is, spin (denoted by the letter I) may have only a certain number of discrete values. The fundamental unit of nuclear spin is Planck's constant (h) divided by 2π, which is denoted by ℏ (h bar). The spins of odd-A nuclei are half integral units of ℏ (i.e.,

$I = 1/2, 3/2, 5/2$, etc. for odd-A nuclei). Even-Z/even-N nuclei have $I = 0$ in their ground state. Odd-Z/odd-N nuclei have spins that are integral multiples of $\hbar$ (i.e., $I = 0, 1, 2, 3$, etc. for odd-Z/odd-N nuclei).

The spin of a proton could be represented by the diagram in Figure 1-1 (small sphere spinning around its own axis). The small magnetic field associated with the "spinning proton" is equivalent to a tiny bar magnet. It is usually referred to as the nuclear magnetic dipole moment (dipole indicating that magnets always possess two poles, usually referred to as a north and a south pole) and is usually denoted by a vector indicating the direction of the field. The direction of the dipole moment is collinear with the axis of rotation.

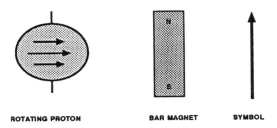

ROTATING PROTON   BAR MAGNET   SYMBOL

FIGURE 1-1. The proton, and other nuclei with a nuclear spin greater than zero, generates a magnetic moment that makes the proton behave like a bar magnet. The magnet has two poles, north (N) and south (S). The magnet is represented as the symbol with a size (magnitude) and a direction indicated by the arrow.

In a glass of water, each water molecule contains two hydrogen atoms. Each hydrogen nucleus can be thought of as a small bar magnet. In the absence of an external magnetic field, the bar magnets are in total disarray. However, if the water is placed in a strong magnetic field, the bar magnets will have a tendency to align with the applied magnetic field (Figure 1-2).

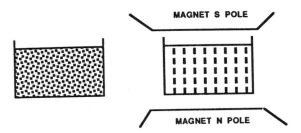

MAGNET S POLE

MAGNET N POLE

FIGURE 1-2. In a container of water (H_2O), the proton magnets are in total disarray. But when the container is placed between the poles of a strong magnet, the proton magnets tend to align with the magnetic field.

It turns out that, for protons, only two alignments (either with or against) are possible in the presence of a magnetic field. This effect can be explained only by using quantum mechanics. For our purposes, it is necessary to know only that the number of alignment states in which a nucleus can exist (in the presence of an applied field) is equal to $(2 \times I) + 1$, where I is the nuclear spin. For the proton, $I = 1/2$, and therefore only two alignment states are possible. The energy difference between the two states (ΔE) is directly proportional to the strength of the applied magnetic field:

$$\Delta E = \gamma B_0$$

where γ is the gyromagnetic ratio of the nucleus (a constant for each NMR-active nucleus) and B_0 is the external magnetic field strength. For the proton, the gyromagnetic ratio is 1.7×10^{-7} eV/T (where eV = electron-volt). Alignment with the field is the lower energy state.

There are a number of different units used to denote magnetic field strength. In the CGS (centimeter-gram-second) system, the basic unit of magnetic field strength is the gauss (G). According to the SI (Système Internationale), the basic unit of magnetic field strength is the tesla (T). One tesla is equal to 10,000 G.

In an external magnetic field of 1.5 T (15,000 G), the energy difference between the two proton alignment states is only 2.6×10^{-7} eV. In radiology, we are accustomed to dealing with energies in the keV range. The energies involved in NMR are one ten-billionth of those used in X-ray radiography and nuclear medicine! This energy range is much different from X-rays and so the unit of energy employed to describe it is different. The frequency of the electromagnetic radiation corresponding to an energy of 2.6×10^{-7} eV is 63.87 MHz. One MHz is equal to 10^6 cycles per second (c/s). This electromagnetic radiation is in the radiofrequency region of the spectrum (the FM radio band is from 88 to 108 MHz).

In terms of frequency, the energy difference between the two alignment states of protons is equal to 42.58 MHz multiplied by B_0, where B_0 is in units of tesla. Since this energy difference is so small, the protons continuously flip back and forth between the two states. However, an equilibrium is established between the two states. At equilibrium, there will be more protons in the lower energy state at any given point in time. However, similar to a chemical equilibrium, individual protons are constantly exchanging between the two states. The size of the plurality depends on the temperature and the magnetic field strength. At 37°C and an external field of 1.5 T, a sample of two million protons would have about ten more protons in the lower energy state (aligned with the field) than the upper energy state (Figure 1-3).

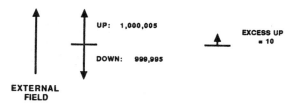

UP: 1,000,005

DOWN: 999,995

EXCESS UP
= 10

EXTERNAL FIELD

FIGURE 1-3. In an external magnetic field, proton magnets align with or against the external field. In this sample of two million protons in a field of 1.5 T, there is a slight excess (ten protons) aligned with the external field.

The essence of the NMR experiment is to send in radiation of the proper frequency which will be absorbed by the protons in a sample. This will occur when the frequency of the radiation is exactly equal to the energy difference between the two alignment states. This frequency is usually referred to as the resonance frequency. The resonance frequency (f_0) is given by

$$f_0 \text{ (MHz)} = 42.58 \times B_0 \text{ (in tesla)}$$

Since for protons at 1.5 T this frequency is near the FM radio range, it is usually referred to as radiofrequency (RF) radiation (or just RF). Since this radiation is applied only for a short time, it is usually called a pulse. Following an RF pulse, the sample of protons is allowed to return to equilibrium. In doing so, the sample emits RF radiation which can be measured.

The distribution of nuclei between two energy states follows the Boltzmann distribution, which is

$$N_{lower}/N_{higher} = \exp(-\Delta E/kT)$$

where N is the number of nuclei in a given state, exp refers to exponentiation in the natural log system (i.e., $\exp(x) = e^x$, where e is the base of the natural logarithms), ΔE is the energy difference between the states, k is the Boltzmann constant (which equals 8.62×10^{-5} eV/K), and T is the temperature in kelvin (K) (equal to temperature in °C + 273).

When ΔE is very small, say 10^{-7} eV, the function $\exp(-\Delta E/kT)$ is very close to e^0, which is 1. The actual value, however, is not quite 1, which leads to a slight excess in the lower energy state (aligned with the external magnetic field). As will be shown in later chapters, it is the excess protons aligned with the main external magnetic field that produce the MRI signal. As field strength increases, the signal strength increases linearly. This is one reason why higher field strength systems yield better images (all other factors being equal). Some examples of the ratio of protons in the two alignment states and the corresponding excess at different field strengths, at 37°C, and for a sample of two million protons are shown below:

| Field Strength | | | Excess # |
Tesla	Gauss	N_{lower}/N_{higher}	Protons
0.15	1,500	1.0000010	0.99
0.35	3,500	1.0000023	2.31
0.50	5,000	1.0000033	3.30
1.00	10,000	1.0000066	6.59
1.50	15,000	1.0000099	9.89
2.00	20,000	1.0000132	13.20
4.00	40,000	1.0000264	26.40

2 Magnetism

The nature of magnetism lies in moving electric charges. It has already been shown that the spinning proton creates a magnetic moment so that it behaves like a simple bar magnet. There are many other examples of magnets in nature. The earth's magnetic field is thought to arise from the rotation of the liquid metal outer core in the interior of the globe. The earth's magnetic field varies from location to location, from about 0.1 G to around 1.0 G. A naturally occurring iron mineral, magnetite (Fe_3O_4) is often magnetic. The magnetism was probably induced by the earth's field as the mineral cooled from the molten state. At mid-ocean rift zones, where molten materials rise, then spread on the sea floor, there is evidence for periodic reversals of the earth's field direction.

In discussions of the magnetic properties of matter, three terms are commonly used: diamagnetism, paramagnetism, and ferromagnetism. These three properties describe the behavior of matter in the presence of an applied magnetic field. If an object is placed in an external magnetic field, the magnetic field inside the object will depend on its magnetic classification as follows: Inside a diamagnetic material, the magnetic field will be slightly less than the external field. For paramagnetic objects, the interior magnetic field will be slightly greater. The magnetic field within a ferromagnetic object will be much greater than the external field. These three properties can be readily explained using the following facts:

1. Moving charged particles generate a magnetic field due to their motion through space.
2. Elementary charged particles possess a fixed intrinsic magnetic field due to spin independent of their motion through space.

All substances will exhibit some degree of diamagnetism. Diamagnetism arises from electrons orbiting nuclei. Every electron within every atom of a substance can therefore be thought of as a tiny electric current loop with an associated magnetic field. Ordinarily, the fields of all of the different electrons are randomly oriented so that the net magnetic field is zero.

It can be shown mathematically that if an external magnetic field is applied to a current loop, the current will change so as to oppose the external field (Lenz's law). Therefore, if we place any substance within an external magnetic field, the orbital motion of the electrons will be altered so as to induce a net magnetic field within the substance that will oppose the external field. In the absence of the external field, the tiny magnetic fields associated with the orbital motion of electrons will be randomly oriented so that there is no net magnetic field. Diamagnetic effects are extremely weak (about two orders of magnitude lower than paramagnetic effects).

Although all substances exhibit diamagnetism, only certain substances exhibit paramagnetism. Paramagnetism arises from electron spin. In most atoms, each electron is paired with an electron of opposite spin so that the magnetic fields associated with these spins cancel out. However, some atoms have unpaired electrons.

When a substance containing atoms with unpaired electrons is exposed to an external magnetic field, the spins of the unpaired electrons will have a tendency to align with the external field. This will cause the substance to attain a net magnetization aligned with the external field. This is referred to as paramagnetism. Therefore, paramagnetism is dominant when a substance contains unpaired electrons.

Certain elements with unpaired electrons will retain their magnetic properties even in the absence of an external magnetic field. This is due to an orderly arrangement of unpaired electron spins in adjacent atoms and is referred to as ferromagnetism. If iron is frozen from the molten state in the presence of a magnetic field, groups of iron atoms form regions in which the atomic magnets are aligned. These regions are called magnetic domains and under a microscope would appear as in Figure 2-1.

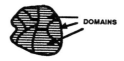

FIGURE 2-1. Magnetic domains in a sample of magnetized iron. The lines indicate the alignment of the iron magnets in each domain.

If the magnets in all of the domains are aligned in the same direction, the iron bar will be maximally magnetized. If the domain alignment is jumbled, the bar is said to be demagnetized. Even the strongest "permanent" magnets lose strength over time, as thermal atomic shaking changes the domain alignments. Japanese scientists have recently developed ferromagnetic alloys (with iron, cobalt, and nickel), containing small amounts of the rare earth metals samarium and europium, that are very strong and more permanent than pure ferromagnetic materials. The most commonly used magnetic alloys are the alnico metals, containing <u>al</u>uminum, <u>ni</u>ckel, and <u>co</u>balt.

Ferromagnetic effects are about six orders of magnitude greater than paramagnetic effects. Ferromagnetic effects can be seen only in macroscopic objects. Individual elementary particles or atoms cannot exhibit ferromagnetism.

Examples of ferromagnetic, paramagnetic, and diamagnetic materials include

Ferromagnetic	Paramagnetic	Diamagnetic
Fe, Co, Ni	Pt, Pr, Sm, Gd	Be, Bi, soft tissue

The strength of magnetic interactions can be precisely quantified by the magnitude of each material's magnetic susceptibility. When an object is placed in an external magnetic field, the field strength inside that object (and even different portions of the same object, if the object is not of uniform consistency) may be different in magnitude from the applied field. The strength of the field inside the object is determined by the magnetic susceptibility of the object, which is defined as the ratio of the field strength inside the object to the applied field strength. A vacuum, for example, has a magnetic susceptibility of one.

3 Electricity and Magnetism

Until 1820, there was no known connection between electricity and magnetism, although the laws describing the two phenomena were known and had many similarities (e.g., like repel, unlike attract, forces inversely proportional to square of distance). One important difference is that electric monopoles exist separately as the negatively charged electron and the positively charged proton. Magnets exist only as dipoles: they always have a north pole and a south pole. If a bar magnet made of iron is broken in half, then in half again, the pieces are themselves always complete magnets and contain both a north pole (N) and a south pole (S). If we continued breaking the magnet, the final piece would of course be an iron atom, which itself acts like a tiny bar magnet.

In 1820, Oersted discovered that direct electric currents produced a magnetic field. Oersted showed that the magnetic field existed only when current flowed (Figure 3-1). The magnetic field lines were oriented in a circular manner around the current-carrying wire. The direction of the circular magnetic field was given by the left thumb rule: if the thumb points in the direction of the electron current flow, the field direction is given by the curling fingers. The south pole is located at the base of the fingers and the north pole is located at the fingertips.

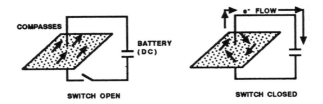

FIGURE 3-1. The Oersted experiment. With no electric current flowing through the circuit, the compass needles point north. When the electric current (electrons) goes through the circuit, a magnetic field is generated around the wire carrying the current.

If the conductor carrying the current is formed into a coil, so that the electron current flows in a series of circles, the magnetic field produced in and around the coil looks exactly like that of a bar magnet, as shown in Figure 3-2. Rather simple coils of four or six turns of superconducting or resistive wires are used to create the main magnetic field for most MRI systems. Several other magnet types exist and are widely used in low- and midfield MRI.

All MRI equipment must provide a source of a strong, constant, and uniform main magnetic field. As previously discussed, moving charge generates a magnetic field. Therefore, as electric current flows through a wire it generates a magnetic field. This field is directed in a circular manner around the wire.

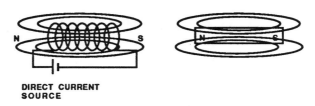

FIGURE 3-2. In the left figure, an electric current flows through the coils, generating a magnetic field that looks exactly like the field of the bar magnet on the right. But there is no ferromagnetic material in the coil.

Suppose a current-carrying wire is formed into a coil, so that the current flows in a series of circles. This arrangement is usually referred to as a solenoid. The solenoid is roughly equivalent to a stack of current rings. The magnetic field within such a solenoid is very uniform at its center. The field strength at the center of a solenoid is directly proportional to the current flowing through the wire and to the number of turns in the coil. If the length of a solenoid is large compared with its width, the field at the center is independent of the width. In addition, the field of such a solenoid remains relatively uniform until one approaches the ends. A solenoid can also be made by using turns of a thin wide ribbon-like conductor.

Most MRI systems use solenoid type coils to generate the main magnetic field. These coils can be resistive or superconducting. In general, the field strength that can be produced using resistive coils is much lower than that produced by super-conducting coils.

Resistive magnets have coils made from conducting metals. The most widely used material is anodized aluminum. The anodizing process creates an insulating layer of aluminum oxide around the conducting metal (Figure 3-3). A ribbon-like anodized aluminum strip is then wound around itself multiple times to form the coil (Figure 3-4).

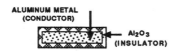

FIGURE 3-3. A cross section of an aluminum conductor that has been anodized. The anodization process produces an insulating layer all around the aluminum. Two pieces of the anodized aluminum placed together would not be in electrical contact.

The strength of the magnetic field obtained in the center of a coil depends on a number of factors, but the most important practical parameters are power going through the coil (watts) and the radius of the coil. The magnetic field (B_0) is proportional to:

$$(W/r\rho)^{1/2}$$

where W is the direct current electric power in watts, r is the inner radius of the coil, and ρ is the resistivity of the coil material. The total resistance (R) of a coil of

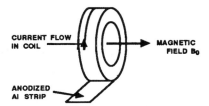

FIGURE 3-4. The creation of a magnetic field by rolling a strip of anodized aluminum into a coil. The process is used to produce resistive magnets, so called because the conductor (aluminum) has an electrical resistance that is not zero.

length L and cross-sectional area A is equal to $\rho L/A$, so that the resistivity is actually the resistance per unit length per unit area.

According to the equation above, the circulating power through the coil must be quadrupled in order to double the magnetic field strength. If the radius of the coil is doubled (e.g., to get larger objects into the magnet), the field strength will fall to 70% of that of the original coil.

It is important to note that the resistivity (ρ) of the coil material is dependent upon temperature. The direct current through the coil (I) is given by Ohm's law: $I = V/R$, where R is the total coil resistance. If R changes, so does I and therefore B_0 as well. The heat produced by the current circulating in the coil is $W = I^2R$. What all this means is that it is best to maintain a constant coil temperature by cooling the coil with water.

Due to power losses and heating of the coil, the maximum field that can be produced in a human body-sized magnet is about 1500 gauss (0.15T). The power required is about 60 kW electrical, and the magnet must remain on continuously to maintain an equilibrium temperature. At 10¢/kWh, the magnet would cost $50,000.00 per year just for electricity.

Low-field permanent magnet systems do offer some advantages. The fringe field surrounding the magnet is so small that magnetic shielding is not required. Life support equipment for anesthetized or severely ill patients may be located at the magnet face with no concern for their proper operation. The accessible space is usually much greater than that of the high-field magnets. The field direction in a permanent magnet is usually vertical (perpendicular to the axis of the bore), which makes it possible to use simpler receiver coils. Against these advantages, low-field systems have a lower signal-to-noise ratio (S/N) compared with high-field systems (S/N is essentially directly proportional to field strength). This requires more signal averages and therefore increased imaging times.

Superconducting magnets use coils made of superconducting materials. By electrical conduction is meant the transport of charged particles through a material. An electric current is defined as the rate of transport (or flow) of charged particles through a conducting material. For a conducting metal wire connected to a battery (or other source of electromotive force), the current is carried by electrons.

For ordinary conductors, a constant supply of a force (i.e., electromotive force) is necessary to move the electrons through the conductor. This need for a force to move the electrons is due the fact that the conductor itself will resist the motion of the electrons through it. This property of resistance is intrinsic to all ordinary conductors. The greater the resistance, the lower the current for a given electromotive force.

When most conducting materials are cooled sufficiently, their resistance to the flow of an electrical current becomes zero. Under these circumstances (of zero resistance), the material is referred to as a superconductor. The temperature below which a given material becomes a superconductor is referred to as the critical temperature (T_c). The property of superconductivity suddenly appears as a material is cooled below the critical temperature. Superconductivity is a strictly quantum mechanical effect and is not easily explained.

Once a material becomes superconducting, a current can flow through it without resistance. Thus, theoretically, once a current is induced to flow through a superconducting material it would continue to flow indefinitely without the need for a source of electromotive force. However, while superconductivity exists only below a critical value for temperature, once a current begins to flow through a superconductor, other factors become important to the superconducting state. These factors are density of current flow (in amperes per square meter) and the magnetic field around the superconductor. The magnetic field within a superconducting material itself is always zero.

There are critical values for current density and magnetic field above which a material will lose its superconductivity (even if its temperature is below the critical temperature). As a current flows through any conductor, it generates a magnetic field around the conductor (the field strength being proportional to the current flow). Therefore, as a current begins to flow through a superconductor, the current itself (through the magnetic field it induces) can result in a loss of superconductivity. Unfortunately, the critical values of current density and magnetic field are quite low for pure superconducting metals so that strong superconducting magnets cannot be constructed from these materials (known as Type I superconductors).

In the 1950s, Type II superconductors were discovered. These materials were alloys of metals such as niobium (Nb), zirconium (Zr), vanadium (V), and titanium (Ti). Unlike Type I superconductors, Type II superconductors have very high critical values for current density and magnetic field. Thus, much stronger magnetic fields can be generated using Type II superconductors.

The most commonly used Type II superconductor is an alloy of niobium and titanium in approximately equal amounts. This alloy is not used as a simple bare wire, but multiple tiny filaments of the alloy are embedded in a matrix of copper to form a wire (Figure 3-5).

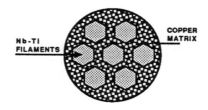

FIGURE 3-5. The arrangement of superconducting filaments in a copper matrix to produce a superconducting wire, which is then wound into a coil or solenoid.

This wire is then wound into a coil configuration. The coil configuration in most magnets uses turns spaced closely together near the ends and spaced further apart near the center of the magnet. When the length of a solenoid is not substantially larger than the width of the coil, this configuration provides a more uniform field than a simple solenoidal arrangement (with the turns evenly spaced).

The major problem of producing a superconducting magnet then becomes maintaining the superconducting material below the critical temperature. The coil is cooled by immersion in liquid helium, which boils at 4.2 K (= –269°C = –452°F). As the liquid boils, it removes heat from the system (from patients, shim coils, RF energy). Cooling designs have evolved over time. For example, the latest General Electric (GE) 1.5-T system uses about 1000 liters (l) of liquid helium, which boils off at a rate of 0.1 l/h. Older designs were more wasteful of the liquid helium, which boiled off at rates of up to 2 l/h. These older systems were significantly more expensive to maintain because liquid helium costs about $5.00/l.

It is not possible to go directly from room temperature to 4.2 K in one step. Older magnet designs consisted of two metal vacuum containers (known as dewars), one inside the other, with the outer container filled with liquid nitrogen (boiling point = 79 K = –194°C = –317°F). Figure 3-6 shows an axial cross section through an older style (Oxford) magnet. In this magnet design, the liquid nitrogen also boils off at about 1 l/h (cost = $0.50/l).

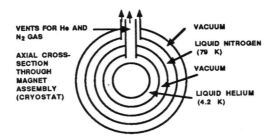

FIGURE 3-6. A cross section through a superconducting magnet of the Oxford design. The system reaches 4.2 K in two stages. The outer dewar contains liquid nitrogen, at 79 K, and the inner dewar holds liquid helium, at 4.2 K. The vacuum chambers between room temperature and the first stage, and between liquid nitrogen and liquid helium, provide thermal insulation.

Newer magnet designs do not use liquid nitrogen. Instead, a helium gas refrigeration system is used for the first cooling stage. The refrigerator is a variant of the system Kammerlingh Onnes used to liquefy helium. The cooled, compressed helium gas is allowed to expand through a small orifice, cooling the gas further. This system causes a washing machine-like noise now heard around MRI magnets. This is the last helium compression stage, just before expansion. A sketch of the newer system is shown in Figure 3-7. The helium gas takes the place of the liquid nitrogen and results in a first-stage cooling to 20 K.

The process of cooling the superconducting coils to below their critical temperature is expensive, but once the current is placed in the coil there is no additional

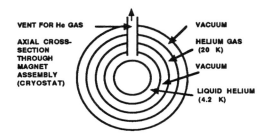

FIGURE 3-7. A cross section through a superconducting magnet of the General Electric design. The system reaches 4.2 K in two stages. The outer dewar is cooled with refrigerated helium gas to about 20 K, and the inner dewar holds liquid helium at 4.2 K. The vacuum chambers between room temperature and the first stage, and between the helium gas and liquid helium, provide thermal insulation.

charge for electricity. But in the newer systems, the cost of operating the helium gas refrigeration system must be considered. Once an electric current is initiated within a superconducting system, the current will circulate forever (and thus create a magnetic field), as long as the temperature of the superconductor remains below the critical temperature (T_c). (There is no electric bill with the older style magnets.)

However, if one part of the coil becomes warm (T_c), heating occurs at that point (as the resistance of the superconducting material becomes nonzero) and the temperature rise spreads rapidly through the remainder of the coil. The circulating currents in high-field magnets range from 250 to 1250 Amperes (A), and this is converted to heat. All of the liquid helium then boils off (and the nitrogen as well in the older style magnets). This is usually referred to as a quench. All magnets are equipped with a "quench button" to do this intentionally in case of a life-threatening emergency where it is imperative to turn off the main magnetic field.

Unfortunately, 1 l of liquid helium or liquid nitrogen becomes approximately 700 l of gas. When a quench occurs, this gas might leak into the magnet room (because the venting system may not be able to handle this large amount of gas) and displace most of the air in the room. This could lead quickly to asphyxiation. Most magnet rooms are equipped with an oxygen sensor set to go off when the oxygen level falls below 18% (from 21% in normal air).

In order to start up the system, an electric current must be initiated within the wire of the superconducting coil. The wires at both ends of a superconducting coil actually penetrate the magnet enclosure and are available as terminals outside of the magnet enclosure. (Obviously, once outside the liquid helium container, this portion of the wire will not be superconducting.) In addition, within the liquid helium container, a superconducting connection between the ends of the wires of the superconducting coil is present. This connection contains a superconducting switch (Figure 3-8). (This switch is made by enclosing a portion of the connection in a material that can be heated from a source outside of the magnet enclosure.)

When the switch becomes superconducting, it creates a short circuit. This connection will bypass those portions of the ends of the superconducting wire outside of the liquid helium container. Therefore, in order to start up the system, a direct current is passed into the superconducting coil (via the outside terminals) until the

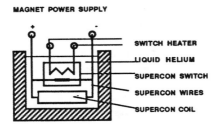

FIGURE 3-8. The superconducting switch that is used to power up a superconducting magnet. The superconducting switch is enclosed in a tube that can be heated to raise its temperature above T_c. Current is sent through the superconducting coil from the magnet power supply. When the desired magnetic field is reached, the heater is turned off, and the switch becomes superconducting.

desired field strength is achieved. At this time, the heater for the superconducting switch is turned off, creating a superconducting short circuit. The external direct current source is also turned off, and as long as the superconducting material is maintained below its critical temperature the same current will flow and the field strength will be maintained at a constant value. Once the appropriate current is started and the system remains cooled, the main magnetic field will persist at relatively constant magnitude for long periods.

A major goal of magnet design is for the field that is produced to be as uniform as possible. Ideally, a perfectly uniform field could be obtained with a uniform current flowing through wires coiled over a sphere, or with an infinitely long sole-noidal coil. Unfortunately, practical magnets are a compromise and their fields will not be perfectly homogeneous, on either the macroscopic or microscopic scale.

In order to compensate for inhomogeneity in the main magnetic field, additional coils are required. These additional coils are called shim coils, which have various shapes, depending on the imperfections for which they are designed to compensate. The strength of the fields required of these coils is rather small since the inhomo-geneities of the main field are small. Ten to twenty shim coils may be required to produce the necessary field homogeneity. All systems use a computer to specify the amount of current necessary in each shim coil. Shim coils may be resistive or superconducting.

As will be discussed later, the MRI process uses the frequency of the measured signal to determine position along the so called frequency-encoding direction (and indirectly, through transient changes in frequency, along the phase-encoding direc-tion). The frequency emitted by a given portion of an object being imaged is directly proportional to the local field strength. It turns out that a change in the strength of the main magnetic field of even a few parts per million can change the position of an object by one pixel or more. Thus, field homogeneity is extremely important. For clinical imaging systems, the required homogeneity is less than about 5 parts per million (ppm). For spectroscopy, the homogeneity should be less than 1 ppm. The homogeneity is often quoted in hertz. A 1.5-T magnet operating at a proton resonance of 63.87 MHz, with a homogeneity of 1 ppm, would be uniform to 64 Hz. The volume of the most homogeneous part of the magnet is about the size of a basketball located at the center of the bore of the magnet.

At points outside of the bore of the magnet, the strength of the magnetic field falls off quickly as the inverse of the cube of the distance from the magnet. Figure 3-9 shows the fringe fields around magnets of various strengths and accessible bores.

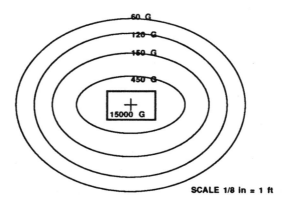

SCALE 1/8 in ≈ 1 ft

FIGURE 3-9. Approximate magnetic field strength around a 1.5-T superconducting magnet.

The following table gives the field limits for interactions with various devices that are affected by magnet fields:

Device	Field Limit (G)
Cathode ray tubes, pacemakers	5
Computers, watches, credit cards	10
Magnetic storage materials	20
Power supplies, spectrometers	50

Figure 3-10 shows the magnetic fields that surround typical imaging magnets, both in the unshielded situation and in a 1.5-T magnet surrounded by 80 tons of steel.

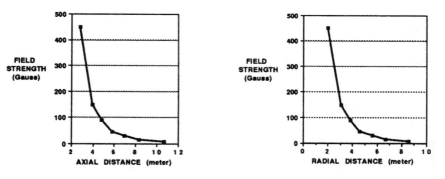

FIGURE 3-10. The variation in the magnetic field around a 1.5-T magnet with a 1-m bore.

A more recent magnetic shield design uses a hexagonal array of steel slabs that surrounds the sides of the magnet, as shown in Figure 3-11.

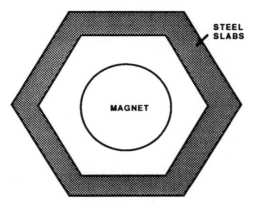

FIGURE 3-11.   A compact magnet shielding design. The steel slabs surrounding the magnet confine the magnetic field.

4 Gradient Coils, RF Coils, and Energy Deposition

Thus far, the components of the imaging system required to generate the main magnetic field have been discussed. There are two other main components of the imaging system: gradient coils and RF coils.

Gradient coils are used to produce nearly uniform changes in the otherwise constant main magnetic field. The gradients are named for the three orthogonal directions of a Cartesian coordinate system: x, y, and z. By convention, the main magnetic field lies along the z direction, the x axis runs from left to right, and the y axis runs from posterior to anterior. Although the gradients are called x, y, and z gradients, the magnetic field changes produced by the gradient coils are in the z direction only. That is, these coils alter the strength of the z magnetic field as a function of position along the x, y, or z axis.

The gradient coils are resistive coils and each have their own power supply and are independently computer controlled. They require large amounts of power (up to 60 kW) and must be rapidly switched on and off hundreds to thousands of times during a typical imaging sequence. The changes in the field strength that they produce are on the order of 0.5 to 1.0 G/cm (5 to 10 mT/m). These coils are mounted on a plastic cylinder (Figure 4-1) inside the bore of the main superconducting magnet. It is the motion (i.e., vibration) of the gradient coils that produces the knocking noise that is characteristic of MRI.

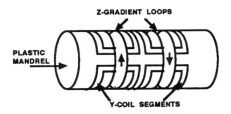

FIGURE 4-1. Two of the three gradient coils of a superconducting magnet. The direct current through the z coil is shown. The direction can be reversed to reverse the gradient magnetic field.

How does this vibration come about? A magnetic field exerts a force on moving charges. As current flows through the gradient coils, the moving charges experience a force. This is manifest as a force on the coil as a whole. As the gradient coil is turned on and off, this force causes it to expand and contract within the plastic cylinder onto which it is mounted. This vibration is the source of the knocking sound. Damping material is used to reduce the sound.

The changing magnetic fields of the gradient coils also interact with all of the other coils in the magnet enclosure and the enclosure itself. This will induce small currents (eddy currents) to flow in the main coil, the shim coils, and the dewars containing the cryogens. These eddy currents in turn produce magnetic fields which may distort the homogeneity of the main magnetic field and the uniformity of the gradients. This problem can be reduced by the use of shielded gradients. Shielded gradient coils consist of two concentric coils: the inner coil produces the desired gradient, while the outer coil is designed to cancel that part of the gradient field that extends into other parts of the magnet.

Space in the magnet bore is reduced by the gradient and shim coils. As shown in Figure 4-2, the original magnet bore diameter has been reduced from 100 cm to about 70 cm.

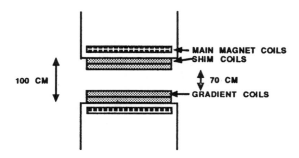

FIGURE 4-2.   The 100-cm diameter of the magnet bore is reduced to 70 cm by the addition of the shim coils and the gradient coils.

In order to perform an MRI experiment, RF excitation pulses are transmitted (at the resonance frequency) to excite the sample. The sample then emits an RF signal that must be received and measured. The transmission of the excitation pulse and the reception of the signal are performed by an RF antenna. This antenna is usually referred to as the RF coil or RF transceiver (transmitter and receiver). A main RF coil is housed within the bore of the magnet and is usually referred to as the body coil. The most commonly used design for a body coil is a so called saddle-shaped coil. This coil actually consists of two identical coils oriented at 90° to one another. This allows these coils to produce circularly polarized RF pulses. Such coils are usually referred to as quadrature coils (Figure 4-3).

In general, there are three types of imaging coils: linear, quadrature, and multi-coil. A linear coil is the simplest type of coil and can be thought of as a single loop of wire (the actual configuration is usually saddle shaped). A quadrature coil can be thought of as two linear coils oriented at 90° to one another. A multicoil consists of multiple linear coils that act independently and simultaneously. Each coil of a multicoil is provided with the capability of reconstructing its own image (unlike the two coils of a quadrature coil, which can only reconstruct a single image).

Quadrature coils use circularly polarized radiation for excitation pulses, and linear coils use linearly polarized radiation for excitation pulses. Circularly polarized pulses give more homogeneous excitation. In addition, quadrature coils have

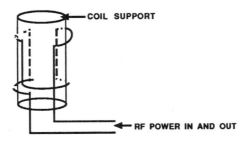

FIGURE 4-3. A saddle coil for transmission and reception of RF radiation.

improved signal-to-noise ratio (S/N) compared with linear coils (by a factor of the square root of 2). Multicoils can be used only in a receive mode.

The same coil used as a transmitter can be used as a receiver. When a quadrature coil is used as a receiver, the signals in each of the component coils must be altered prior to signal processing. Since quadrature coils are oriented at 90° to one another, their signals will be phase shifted by 90°. After phase shifting one of the signals back by 90° (such that the signals are once again in phase), the signals from each of the coils can then be added prior to signal processing. The addition of the signals results in an improvement of the S/N (compared with a linear coil acting as a receiver) by a factor of the square root of 2.

It is important to note that a circularly polarized RF pulse is not required to produce excitation. As long as the time variation of a pulse (i.e., the frequency) is at the resonance frequency, it will cause excitation. However, circularly polarized radiation does provide a more uniform and more energy efficient means of excitation.

There is a great deal of art, and some science, that goes into the design of the RF coil. The objective of coil design is efficiency and uniformity in radiating and detecting RF signal power. In order to excite the protons within a sample in the coil, the RF energy must be delivered in a way that causes the protons that are aligned with the main magnetic field to be tipped away from the main field direction. This process will be discussed in greater detail in later chapters. For now, suffice it to say that the purpose of the RF coil is to create an oscillating magnetic field, called the B_1 field, that is applied across the sample and at right angles to the main magnetic field, B_0.

1   ENERGY DEPOSITION

At 1.5 T, the resonance frequency of water protons is 63.87 MHz. By applying a source of alternating current across the terminals of the RF coil, a time-varying magnetic field is produced. Alternating current is produced by an RF power supply. These are commercially available and are used by commercial radio stations and ham operators. The power in watts required to excite the protons in the body depends on the size (mass and volume) of the object being imaged. Typical power levels are 4 kW for heads and up to 16 kW for bodies.

In its original approval of MRI systems, the Food and Drug Administration (FDA) set limits on the power that could be delivered to patients during MRI. The limit was set in terms of the rate of power deposition, defined as watts per kilogram. The unit is more commonly known as the specific absorption rate (SAR). Analysis of the units of SAR shows that it is a measure of energy delivered to a mass per unit time: joules (J) per kilogram per second (1 W = 1 J/s).

The metabolic heat produced by an awake, resting adult human is about 1.5 W/kg. During a tennis match, the metabolic rate increases to about 7.5 W/kg, and world-class sprinters can produce more than 20 W/kg during a 60-m dash. The limit set by the FDA for the SAR during MRI is 0.4 W/kg, averaged over the whole body, and further averaged over a time period of 0.1 h (6 min).

Part of the system software in MRI devices is used to calculate the SAR, based on the patient's weight and the following imaging parameters: the number of sections imaged per study, the number of spin echoes obtained in each section, the total imaging time, the repetition time (TR), the section thickness, the pulse sequence (gradient echo sequences usually have very low SARs), the resolution desired (matrix size), and, finally, whether saturation pulses are used.

Many MRI procedures in the body can easily exceed the average SAR limit of 0.4 W/kg. Lower power levels are used in the head coil and the extremity coil (up to about 4 kW), and the FDA allows the power to be averaged over the total body mass. As a result, average SARs in head or extremity studies are well below 0.4 W/kg. The average SAR limit of 0.4 W/kg is a significant limitation on MRI scans, which require the use of the body coil as a transmitter or transceiver.

In November 1988, the FDA revised the standards for MRI devices, recognizing that the effects of RF heating were more important than the average SAR itself. The revised FDA recommendations retain the SAR limit of 0.4 W/kg, but allow any SAR as long as the following conditions are met:

1. The maximum increase in body core temperature does not exceed +1°C (1.8°F).
2. The maximum temperature produced in the head does not exceed 38°C (100.4°F).
3. The maximum temperature produced in the trunk does not exceed 39°C (102.2°F).
4. The maximum temperature produced in the extremities does not exceed 40°C (104°F).

As will be shown later, these maxima are unlikely to be exceeded in any scan sequence. In addition to the average SAR limit, the FDA has also specified that the maximum SAR delivered to any 1 g of tissue not exceed 8 W/kg — the "peak" SAR. A number of studies have shown that there is no evidence for "hot spots" during MRI. This is not too surprising, since the wavelength of the radiation used for MRI at 1.5 T is several meters, and even longer for lower field strength magnets.

The FDA limits on SAR were adopted in their entirety from the American National Standards Institute (ANSI) (known as the ANSI-82 standards). The ANSI-82 standards are intended to apply to chronic exposure of the general population (both occupational and nonoccupational) and not to purposeful exposure of patients. In fact both diathermy and cancer hyperthermia procedures exceed the ANSI-82 standard by a factor of ten. More recently, the National Council on Radiation Protection and Measurements (NCRP) has recommended that the limiting whole-body average SAR for occupational workers be 0.4 W/kg, *but* 0.08 W/kg for the general public (NCRP report no. 86).

The general consensus of numerous experiments conducted on animals and limited, retrospective epidemiological studies on humans (e.g., the U.S. embassy personnel exposed in Moscow) is that there are no significant biological effects from exposure to RF radiation. However, most experimental studies have been performed at microwave oven frequencies (2450 MHz = 2.45 GHz), and their applicability to the MRI frequency range of 1 to 100 MHz has been questioned.

In addition to the excitation of proton spins in selected locations in the body, the RF pulse interacts with the body by inducing voltage or current loops in the outer layers of the body. These currents are produced in the tissues by the B_1 magnetic field of the RF pulse.

A simple worst-case calculation can be performed to estimate the heating effect of RF on the body. For the calculation, the following assumptions are made:

1. SAR = 2 W/kg
2. Tissue-specific heat = 0.83 kcal/kg/°C.
3. 1 kcal = 4186 J (W-s).
4. Scan time = 20 minutes = 1200 seconds.
5. Normal thermoregulatory response is absent.

$$\Delta \text{Temperature} = \frac{\text{SAR}\,(\text{W/kg}) \times \text{time (s)}}{4186\,\text{W-s/kcal} \times 0.83\,\text{kcal/kg/}°\text{C}}$$

$$= \frac{\text{SAR}\,(\text{W/kg}) \times \text{time (s)}}{3474\,\text{W-s/kg/}°\text{C}}$$

For the parameters as given above:

$$\Delta \text{Temperature} = \frac{2 \times 1200}{3474} = 0.7°\text{C}$$

This quick calculation on a system that has no thermoregulatory response may be compared to the temperature changes experienced in day-to-day living. Normal diurnal temperature variations in humans are about ±1°C from the set point of 37°C. Thus, it seems unlikely that the heating effect of MRI could cause any acute effects in healthy humans. Healthy people with normal thermoregulatory response can dissipate excess metabolic (or deposited) heat by increasing their peripheral blood flow and/or sweating. The former response would require an increase in cardiac output of perhaps 20%. This could present a problem to patients with compromised cardiac performance, although there has never been a reported incident of this nature in MRI.

2   SCAN PREPARATION

Once the appropriate coil is selected, the patient is placed on the scanner table and a landmark is established. A dual-laser light is activated which projects two lines onto the patient: one line parallel to the table top at the level of isocenter and a second line perpendicular to the table top. The area of interest is positioned so that these lines are at its center. The level selected is then used as a reference for the remainder of the examination. All positions in the superior/inferior (S/I), anterior/posterior (A/P), and left/right (L/R) directions are given with respect to landmark. The center of the landmark is at S0(I0), A0(P0), L0(R0) by definition. The operator and computer system then directs the patient table to be moved to the center of the magnet bore, where the homogeneity is best.

Before the actual scanning process can begin a **prescan** process must be completed. On most imaging systems, the prescan process can be done automatically or manually. The prescan process typically consists of four steps:

- A coarse center frequency adjustment
- A flip angle adjustment
- A fine center frequency adjustment
- A receive gain setting adjustment

The resonance frequency of the protons at the image locations in each patient will be slightly different (with differences in the kilohertz range) due to slight differences in magnetic susceptibility. The first step of the prescan process determines the resonance frequency of protons at the center of the imaging volume. In essence, the machine must match the transmitter resonance frequency to the received resonance frequency. The presence of the patient within the scanner also alters slightly the resonance frequency of the transmitter coil, which then has to be adjusted.

The second step of the prescan process is to determine the energy of a so called 90° pulse. This is done by applying excitation pulses in a sequential step-wise fashion and measuring the received signal after each pulse. The initial pulse is of a low energy (well below that required for a 90° pulse). As pulses of higher energy are sequentially applied, the received signal will steadily rise until a peak is reached, after which the received signal will fall. By definition, a 90° pulse will give maximal received signal. Therefore, the energy that gave maximal signal *is* a 90° pulse.

This same process is also used to determine the energy of a 180° pulse. Theoretically, if an RF pulse of amplitude A applied for time T gives a 90° pulse, then an RF pulse of amplitude 2A applied for time T (or an RF pulse of amplitude A applied for time 2T) would give a 180° pulse. The machine actually verifies the precise values of amplitude and duration of the RF pulse by applying pulses near the theoretical value until no signal is received. A 180° pulse should produce no signal because no transverse magnetization is created.

The third step of the prescan process is a repeat of the first, with a finer center frequency determined.

The fourth step of the prescan process determines the **gain** settings of the receiver electronics. The actual received signal is quite weak and is electronically amplified.

The gain is the degree of amplification of the signal prior to its being processed. Due to memory limitations of the signal processor, the amplified signal must not exceed a certain maximal value (S_{max}). The gain settings are adjusted such that the maximal intensity of the amplified signal is less than S_{max} (typically 50% to 85% is chosen).

It is important to note that the prescan process is performed only for one section of tissue of the prescribed volume to be imaged (usually the center section). This is why the 50–85% value is used. In case the noncenter sections have higher signal structures than the center section, this provides a safety margin.

Once the prescan process is completed, scanning can be initiated. The prescan process is usually performed prior to each acquisition. This process is time consuming, requiring 1 to 2 min to perform, if done automatically, and longer if done manually.

5 The Behavior of Protons in a Magnetic Field

The behavior of protons placed in a magnetic field is similar to the behavior of a spinning top placed in the gravitational field of the earth. A spinning top is simply an object with mass that rotates about its own axis. Just as an object that moves in a straight line has linear momentum (equal to mass multiplied by linear velocity), an object that spins will have an associated angular momentum. Whereas linear momentum is directed along the line of motion of an object, angular momentum is directed along the line around which the object rotates (Figure 5-1). For a spinning top, the angular momentum is directed along the axis of the top.

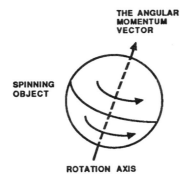

FIGURE 5-1. A spinning object generates an angular momentum, a vector quantity that has both magnitude and direction. The direction is along the line of the axis of rotation.

If not spinning, a top that is placed on its tip will simply fall over due to the effects of gravity. If spinning rapidly, the top will initially remain upright when placed on its tip. In this position, the axis of the top (and therefore its angular momentum) will be perfectly aligned with the gravitational field of the earth (Figure 5-2). Due to frictional forces, the top will spin more slowly over time. As it slows down, the top will begin to tip over such that the axis of the top is no longer aligned with the gravitational field of the earth. When this occurs, it can be shown mathematically that the force of gravity exerts a torque on the spinning top and changes its angular momentum such that the top rotates about the axis of the gravitational field (Figure 5-3). This rotational motion is usually referred to as precession. Precessional motion will occur as long as the top continues to spin about its own axis. The frequency of the precessional motion is inversely proportional to the angular momentum of the top (i.e., the slower the top spins, the faster is the rate of precession) and directly proportional to the gravitational field strength.

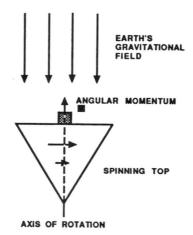

FIGURE 5-2. The axis of rotation of a spinning top and its angular momentum vector are aligned with the gravitational field of the earth.

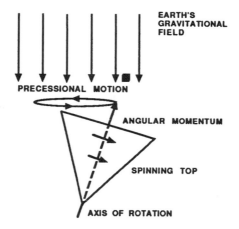

FIGURE 5-3. As the spinning of the top slows, the gravitational force changes the angular momentum. The top starts to wobble, or precess. The rate of precession depends on the angular momentum and the strength of the gravitational force.

As noted previously, protons (and other elementary particles) possess an intrinsic spin and are therefore equivalent to tiny spinning magnetic tops. Due to their spin, these particles possess an intrinsic angular momentum. When they are placed in an external magnetic field, they behave in a manner identical to a spinning top placed in a gravitational field. As long as the angular momentum of the particles remains aligned with the axis of the external field, they will "spin" undisturbed. However, if this alignment is disturbed, the external magnetic field exerts a torque on the protons and they will precess about the axis of the external field. Unlike the spinning top (which slows due to frictional forces), the spin of protons is an intrinsic property that persists forever. Therefore, as long as they are exposed to an external magnetic field and are not aligned along the magnetic field, the protons will precess about the axis of the field.

Analogous to the spinning top, the frequency of precession of a proton in the presence of an external field is inversely proportional to its angular momentum and directly proportional to the external field strength. Since the angular momentum of a proton is a fixed intrinsic quantity (which can be predicted only by quantum mechanics), the frequency of precession is directly proportional to the applied external field. The constant of proportionality is called the gyromagnetic ratio γ. Therefore, if protons are exposed to a field of strength B, they will precess at a frequency of γB. The value of γB is such that at 1.5 T, protons will precess at a frequency of approximately 63.87 MHz.

What actually happens when a collection of protons is subjected to an external magnetic field? The effect can be described in terms of individual protons (which requires concepts of quantum mechanics) or in terms of the effect on the collection as a whole (which requires only classical mechanics).

Using quantum mechanics, it can be shown that individual protons can assume only one of two possible orientations when placed in an external magnetic field (B_0). These are shown in Figure 5-4. Although these allowed orientations are usually described as being with or against the external field, they are not actually directly along the axis of the external field. As a result, the protons will precess around the axis of B_0.

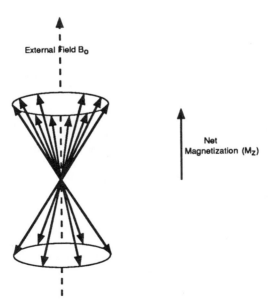

FIGURE 5-4. A collection of protons in an external magnetic field, with about half aligned with, and about half aligned against, the external field. There is a small excess of protons aligned with the field, producing a net magnetization (M_z) along the external field direction.

It is energetically more favorable for a proton to be oriented with the external field. The energy difference between the two allowed orientations is directly proportional to the strength of the applied magnetic field. Even at a field strength of 1.5 T, this energy difference is small. In fact, at body temperature, the energy of thermal motion greatly exceeds this difference, so protons are constantly exchanging between the two allowed orientations. Over time, however, the protons will achieve an equilibrium such that at any instant there is a net excess aligned with the external field (the energetically more favorable state). This occurs even though individual protons are still constantly exchanging between the two states. This is exactly analogous to a chemical equilibrium.

Therefore, a collection of protons in an external magnetic field can be thought of as consisting of two separate populations of spinning magnetic tops: one population aligned somewhat along the external field and the second aligned somewhat opposite the external field, with protons in both populations precessing around the axis of the external field (Figure 5-4). When equilibrium is achieved, the small net excess of protons aligned with the field causes the sample to obtain a net magnetization in the direction of the external field. In addition, the precessional motion of the individual protons causes them to be randomly distributed around the axis of the external field. This random distribution results in zero net magnetization in the plane perpendicular to the external field. Thus, at equilibrium, the net magnetization of a collection of protons points along the direction of the external field even though the magnetization of each individual proton is at an angle with respect to this field.

At 1.5 T and at body temperature, the net excess of protons aligned along the external field at equilibrium will amount to approximately five per million. Although this seems like a small amount, 18 g (1 mol) of water contains Avogadro's number (6.02×10^{23}) of individual water molecules (with each water molecule containing two protons).

When a collection of protons (such as a patient) is initially placed in an external magnetic field, the time required to achieve equilibrium depends on the tissue type and whether the protons are in water or lipid. The **T1 relaxation time** of a tissue is a measure of the time required to reach equilibrium alignment with the external field. The larger the T1 value, the longer the time required to reach equilibrium. That is, the larger the T1 value of a tissue, the longer it takes for protons to align with an external field. The reciprocal of the T1 relaxation time is the **T1 relaxation rate (R1)**. That is, R1 = 1/T1. The larger the value of T1, the smaller the value of R1, and the slower the relaxation rate.

By convention, magnetization along the direction of the applied magnetic field is referred to as **longitudinal** magnetization and magnetization in the plane perpendicular to the external field is referred to as **transverse** magnetization. Also by convention, when using a Cartesian coordinate system, the direction of the external field is defined as the z axis and the transverse plane as the plane formed by the x and y axes.

Disregarding the behavior of the individual protons, then, the effect of an external magnetic field on a collection of protons is to create a net magnetization within the collection. This net magnetization is precisely along the direction of the external field. Unless it is disturbed by other external influences, the net magnetization will remain constant in both magnitude and direction. The net magnetization suffices to accurately describe the collection of protons (Figure 5-4).

For discussion purposes, it is easier to explain some phenomena in terms of the behavior of the individual protons, whereas other phenomena are easier to explain in terms of the behavior of the net magnetization. However, in order to explain the behavior of the net magnetization of a collection of protons, it is important to note that the net magnetization will itself possess the property of spin. This results from the fact that the net magnetization is derived from individual protons each of which possesses spin. At equilibrium, the net magnetization is aligned along the direction of the external field and therefore does not precess. If, however, something disturbs the alignment of the net magnetization, it will precess around the axis of the external field (Figure 5-5). This is the key to understanding the origin of the MR signal.

Suppose the external magnetic field is of strength B_0 and is oriented along the positive z axis of a Cartesian coordinate system. If a collection of protons is placed within this field, then at equilibrium the net magnetization will be oriented along the positive z axis. Suppose the net magnetization is disturbed such that it no longer lies along the z axis. Due to its spin, it will then precess around the z axis in a clockwise manner. The frequency of precession (ω_0) will be equal to γB_0. This is usually referred to as the resonance frequency.

Suppose we view the rotating net magnetization from a coordinate system [denoted by (x′,y′,z′)] that itself rotates clockwise around the z axis at frequency ω_0. In this coordinate system, the net magnetization (as well as the individual protons) will be stationary. It is as if the main magnetic field strength (B_0) in this rotating coordinate system is zero (because there is no precessional motion) (Figure 5-6).

Now suppose a second weak external magnetic field (of strength B_1) is applied. Furthermore, suppose this field lies within the xy plane and rotates clockwise around the z axis at frequency ω_0 (i.e., at the frequency of rotation of the net magnetization and individual protons). The B_1 field will be stationary in the rotating coordinate system. For simplicity, let us assume that it lies along the y′ axis of the rotating coordinate system.

Due to its intrinsic spin, the net magnetization will now precess around the axis of the B_1 field (i.e., around the y′ axis). The rate of this rotation will be equal to γB_1. In general, $B_1 \ll B_0$. If such a field is applied for a short period of time, its effect will be to slowly rotate the net magnetization toward the transverse plane (Figure 5-7). Whereas the motion appears very simple in the rotating coordinate system, in the original nonrotating (x,y,z) coordinate system, the motion is much more complex. In the (x,y,z) system, the net magnetization is rapidly rotating around the z axis and at the same time very slowly rotating around the axis of the B_1 field.

The degree of rotation caused by the B_1 field is usually denoted by the number of degrees of rotation of the net magnetization away from the positive z axis. For example, a 90° rotation corresponds to a rotation of the net magnetization into the transverse (i.e., xy) plane. A 180° rotation corresponds to a rotation of the net magnetization to a position along the negative z axis (Figure 5-7C).

Suppose the net magnetization is viewed in a coordinate system that rotates clockwise around the z axis at a rate less than ω_0 (say $\omega_0 - \Delta\omega$). In this coordinate

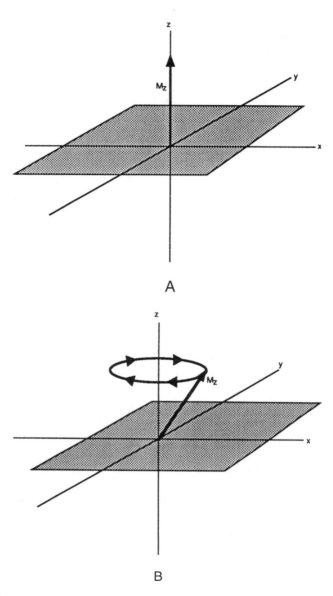

FIGURE 5-5. (A) As long as the net magnetization lies along the z axis, it remains stationary. (B) When the net magnetization, M_z, is disturbed so that it no longer lies along the z axis, it starts to undergo a precessional motion around the z axis. The precessional motion is caused by the external magnetic field.

system, the net magnetization will be precessing in a clockwise direction around the z axis at a rate equal to $\Delta\omega$. This means that the effective strength of the B_0 field within this coordinate system (denoted by B) must be such that $\Delta\omega = \gamma B$. That is, $B = \Delta\omega/\gamma$. This field is still oriented along the positive z axis because the precessional

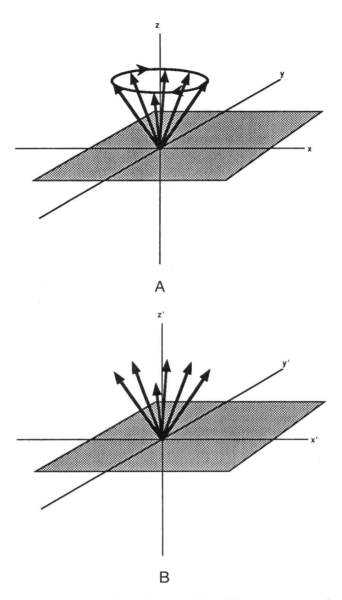

FIGURE 5-6. Two ways of looking at the precession of the proton magnets in the external field. (A) In a fixed plane of reference, the protons precess around the z axis. (B) In a rotating reference frame (denoted by primed coordinates), the protons do not appear to have any motion.

motion is clockwise around the z axis. (In a coordinate system rotating clockwise at a rate $\omega_0 + \Delta\omega$, the net magnetization would be rotating in a counterclockwise direction at a rate $\Delta\omega$. In this case the effective main field would be of strength $\Delta\omega/\gamma$, but would be oriented along the negative z axis.)

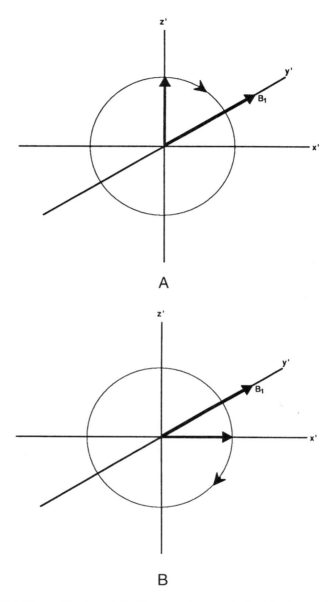

FIGURE 5-7. The application of the B_1 external magnetic field in the rotating frame. B_1 is in the $x'y'$ plane and along the y' axis. In (A), the B_1 field has just been turned on. Depending upon the strength and time of application, the B_1 field will cause a rotation of the net magnetization. In (B), there has been a 90° rotation.

Return now to the coordinate system that rotates clockwise around the z axis at a rate $\omega_0 - \Delta\omega$. The effective main magnetic field in this coordinate system is of magnitude $\Delta\omega/\gamma$ and is oriented along the positive z axis. As above, suppose a second

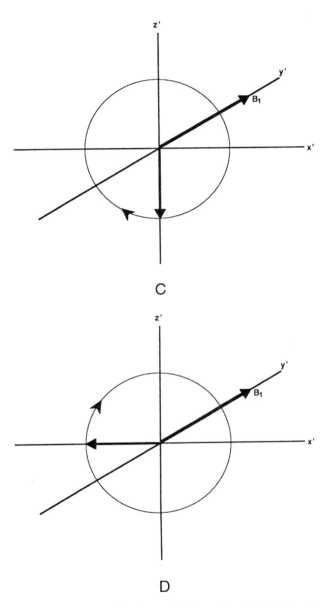

FIGURE 5-7 C&D. In (C), there has been a 180° rotation. In (D), there has been a 270° rotation.

external magnetic field (of strength B_1) is applied. Furthermore, suppose this field lies within the xy plane and rotates clockwise around the z axis at frequency $\omega_0 - \Delta\omega$. The B_1 field will be stationary in the rotating coordinate system. For simplicity, assume that it lies along the y′ axis of the rotating coordinate system.

The effective main magnetic field is not zero in this new rotating coordinate system. Therefore, the field experienced by the net magnetization in this coordinate system is the vector sum of B and B_1. Now B lies along the positive z axis and B_1 lies along the y' axis. The net applied field therefore lies somewhere between these two. The net magnetization of the collection of protons will therefore precess around this net magnetic field. Its motion is therefore determined by the orientation of this net field (Figure 5-8).

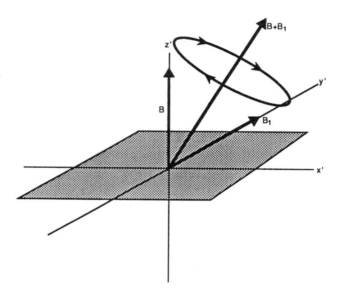

FIGURE 5-8. The net magnetic field lies between B and B_1. This causes the net magnetization, M_z, to rotate around this magnetic field.

If $B \gg B_1$, then the net field will be almost along the positive z axis. In that case, the net magnetization will essentially precess around the z axis. It was already doing this prior to application of the B_1 field. Therefore, in this case, the B_1 field has an almost negligible effect and will not cause the net magnetization to rotate into the xy plane. On the other hand, if $B_1 \gg B$, then the field will be almost along the y' axis. In this case, the net magnetization will essentially precess around the y' axis. Therefore, if $B_1 \gg B$, the B_1 field is very effective in causing the net magnetization to rotate into the xy plane.

Now the magnitude of B is strictly determined by $\Delta\omega$. If $\Delta\omega = 0$, then $B = 0$ and $B_1 \gg B$. In this case, even a weak B_1 field rotating around the z axis at frequency ω_0 will be effective in rotating the net magnetization into the transverse plane. If $\Delta\omega$ is large, then the B_1 field would have to be very strong to rotate the net magnetization into the transverse plane. Therefore, for a fixed strength of the B_1 field, it will be most effective in rotating the net magnetization into the transverse plane when the B_1 field itself rotates clockwise around the z axis at the resonance frequency ω_0.

Thus far, only the effects of the B_1 field on the net magnetization of the sample have been discussed. The B_1 field results in a simple rotation of the net magnetization of the sample. However, what is the effect of the B_1 field upon individual protons within the sample? As noted previously, in order to discuss the motion of the individual protons, we must resort to quantum mechanics.

From a quantum mechanical point of view, an individual proton has two attributes. These are alignment with respect to the B_0 field (which is either with or against) and rotation around the axis of the B_0 field. The net longitudinal magnetization of a sample of protons is strictly determined by the difference in the number of protons aligned with or against the applied field. If more protons are aligned with the B_0 field, there will be a net longitudinal magnetization aligned with the B_0 field. If more protons are aligned against the B_0 field, then there will be a net longitudinal magnetization aligned against the B_0 field. If there are an equal number of protons in each orientation, then there will be zero net longitudinal magnetization.

The net transverse magnetization within a sample is strictly determined by the distribution of individual protons around the axis of the B_0 field as they rotate. If the individual protons are randomly distributed around the axis of the B_0 field, then there will be zero net transverse magnetization. If the individual protons are not randomly distributed around the axis of the B_0 field but somehow rotate together (i.e., in phase), then the net transverse magnetization will not be zero and it will itself rotate around the axis of the B_0 field (Figure 5-9).

What is the effect of a 90° rotation by the B_1 field described above? The complete loss of longitudinal magnetization is exactly equivalent to causing the number of protons aligned with the B_0 field to equal the number of protons aligned against the B_0 field. In addition, the creation of transverse magnetization is exactly equivalent to causing the individual protons to rotate somewhat together (i.e., in phase) around the axis of the B_0 field.

Thus, the effect of the transient application of the B_1 field is to disturb the equilibrium distribution of the individual protons with respect to their alignment along the B_0 field (with or against) and with respect to rotational distribution around the axis of the B_0 field (random or relatively in phase).

From the quantum mechanical point of view, the rotating B_1 field is exactly equivalent to the magnetic field of electromagnetic radiation at a frequency equal to the rotational frequency of the B_1 field. Recall that as a wave phenomenon, electromagnetic radiation consists of time-varying electric and magnetic fields. As a particulate phenomenon, electromagnetic radiation consists of photons of energy directly proportional to the frequency of the radiation. The constant of proportionality is equal to Planck's constant (i.e., the energy of a photon of frequency ν is equal to $h\nu$). Thus, from the point of view of quantum mechanics, photons (in the form of electromagnetic radiation) provide the necessary energy to disturb the equilibrium distribution of the individual protons within a collection of protons placed in the B_0 field.

What is the actual strength of the B_1 field used in clinical imaging? Denote the frequency of rotation of the net magnetization around the B_1 field as f. Then, f = γB_1, where γ is the gyromagnetic ratio. The gyromagnetic ratio for the proton is

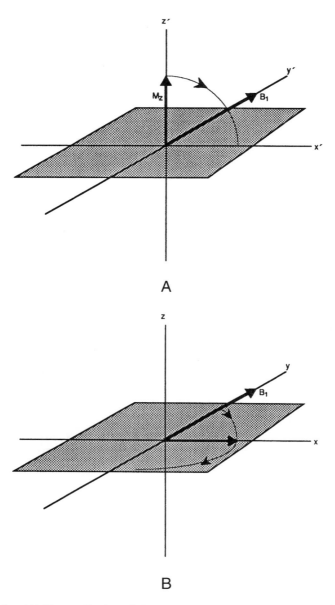

FIGURE 5-9. (A) The application of the B_1 external magnetic field in the rotating frame causes the M_z to rotate slowly into the transverse (xy) plane. A 90° rotation is shown here. (B) The transverse magnetization created will then precess around the z axis.

4258 Hz/G. Recall that frequency is in units of cycles (or rotations) per second (Hz) and that magnetic field strength is in units of gauss. On most imaging systems, the B_1 field is turned on for a short but fixed period of time. If the B_1 field is turned on for t seconds, then the net magnetization will undergo f × t rotations. Since a 90°

rotation corresponds to one-quarter of a cycle, we require that $f \times t = (\gamma B_1) \times t = 1/4$. Therefore, $B_1 = 1/4\gamma t$. On the GE Signa 1.5-T system, $t = 3.2$ ms. Therefore, $B_1 = 0.018$ G.

Let us summarize the discussion to this point. A collection of protons is placed into a strong external magnetic field (B_0), which is oriented along the positive z axis of a Cartesian coordinate system. The individual protons will equilibrate into two populations precessing (at frequency $\omega_0 = \gamma B_0$) around the z axis, one population aligned somewhat along the positive z axis and the other aligned somewhat along the negative z axis. At equilibrium, there will be a small net excess of protons in the population aligned along the positive z axis. This results in a net longitudinal magnetization along the positive z axis. Both populations of protons will precess around the z axis and at equilibrium they will be randomly distributed around the z axis.

Exposing a sample of protons to a weak external magnetic field that itself rotates clockwise at frequency ω_0 around the z axis causes the net magnetization to rotate slowly (at a rate equal to γB_1) into the xy plane. At the same time, the net magnetization will be precessing around the z axis at the rate ω_0. If the B_1 field rotates around the z axis at a frequency other than ω_0, it will be much less effective in rotating the net magnetization into the transverse plane. The effect of the rotating B_1 field is to convert longitudinal magnetization into transverse magnetization. The degree of conversion is determined by the strength and duration of the B_1 field. Once again, a 90° rotation completely converts longitudinal magnetization into transverse magnetization.

When net transverse magnetization is created by applying an external rotating magnetic field, the net transverse magnetization (which possesses spin) will itself rotate in the xy plane at the resonance frequency (i.e., 63.87 MHz at 1.5 T). It is this time-varying magnetic field that generates the MR signal. This rotating magnetic field induces voltage changes within a receiver coil of the MR scanner. The frequency of the detected signal would therefore be at 63.87 MHz. That is, the frequency of the signal emitted by the rotating transverse magnetization is equal to the frequency of rotation.

In general, when performing an MRI experiment, the rotating magnetic field (B_1 field) is applied only for a short period of time and is referred to as a pulse (a pulse being something of short duration). Since the frequency of rotation of the B_1 field is the same frequency as radio waves, it is also commonly referred to as an RF pulse. The most commonly used RF pulse is the 90° pulse. If, for example, a 90° pulse has been applied to a collection of protons, then immediately after it is turned off there will be zero longitudinal magnetization and maximal transverse magnetization. However, what happens after the RF pulse is turned off?

After all external influences have been removed, the system of protons will always return to the equilibrium situation. Therefore, longitudinal magnetization will begin to steadily increase until it reaches its initial value oriented along the positive z axis. The rate of return to equilibrium will vary from tissue to tissue, depending on their T1 values.

As discussed later, when an MRI experiment is performed, the sample is excited by RF pulses many times at fixed time intervals. If these intervals were long enough, then all tissues (regardless of their T1 value) would completely recover their longitudinal magnetization prior to the next excitation. In such a case, the signal emitted by a given tissue would be relatively independent of T1 effects. However, if the time between excitations is not long (compared to T1), then the amount of longitudinal magnetization present at the time of each sequential excitation will vary from tissue to tissue (depending on T1). In fact, for several types of imaging sequences, several RF pulses are applied at the excitation interval before signal measurements are begun. This establishes an equilibrium state (or steady state) prior to the imaging process.

What happens to the transverse magnetization that is created by the application of an RF pulse? As long as transverse magnetization persists, a signal will be detected. Once again, the system will return to the equilibrium situation. Recall that at equilibrium, the net transverse magnetization is zero because all of the protons are randomly distributed around the z axis. Once an RF pulse is turned off, the protons will rapidly get out of phase (i.e., they will return to a random distribution around the z axis) and the transverse magnetization created by the RF pulse will decay to zero.

The **T2** relaxation time of a tissue is a measure of how long transverse magnetization (created by an RF pulse) persists once the RF pulse is turned off (i.e., how long the protons continue to precess in phase once the RF pulse is turned off). The longer the T2 relaxation time, the longer the transverse magnetization persists. This process is independent of T1. The reciprocal of the T2 relaxation time is the T2 relaxation rate (R2). That is, $R2 = 1/T2$. In general, for any given tissue, $T1 \gg T2$ (which is equivalent to $R2 \gg R1$). That is, for most tissues, the rate of loss of transverse magnetization greatly exceeds the rate of recovery of longitudinal magnetization. It is important to remember, however, that these are independent properties.

Before discussing the imaging process, one more diversion is required. In the discussion above, a rotating magnetic field was used to tip the net magnetization. How is such a field generated? If a constant direct current is passed through a wire, it generates a magnetic field of constant magnitude and direction. This does not imply that the field is the same at all points in space, only that the strength and direction at each point in space does not change over time. By passing a direct current through a saddle-shaped wire (coil) whose long axis is along the z axis, a magnetic field can be generated in the xy plane. The direction of the field can be changed by simply rotating the coil.

Suppose a saddle-shaped coil is oriented to produce a field along the x direction. If an alternating current is passed through the coil, the magnitude of the field along the x axis will change as a function of time. Suppose the alternating current is sinusoidal in nature, and suppose the strength of the field along the x axis as a function of time is given by $B_1\cos2\pi\omega_0 t$. A positive strength indicates the field points along the positive x axis and a negative strength indicates that the field points along the negative x axis. Then at time $t = 0$, since $\cos0° = 1$, the field will point along the positive x axis and be of magnitude B_1. At time $t = 1/4\omega_0$, the field is zero. At time $t = 1/2\omega_0$, the field will point along the negative x axis and be of magnitude B_1. At time $t = 3/4\omega_0$, the field will be zero. At time $t = 1/\omega_0$, the field will once again point along the positive x axis and be of magnitude B_1. Thus, the field strength along the x axis will cycle every $1/\omega_0$ seconds (i.e., it will be of frequency ω_0).

Suppose a second saddle coil is rotated 90° from the coil above so that its field is along the y axis. In addition, suppose an alternating current passed through this coil has the form $B_1\sin2\pi\omega t$. Then at time $t = 0$, the field will be zero along the positive y axis. At time $t = 1/4\omega_0$, the field will point along the positive y axis and be of magnitude B_1. At time $t = 1/2\omega_0$, the field will be zero. At time $t = 3/4\omega_0$, the field will point along the negative y axis and be of magnitude B_1. At time $t = 1/\omega_0$, the field will once again be zero. Thus, the field strength along the y axis will cycle every $1/\omega_0$ seconds (i.e., it will have frequency ω_0).

If currents are passed through both of the coils simultaneously, the net magnetic field within the xy plane will be the sum of the two fields. This is a vector sum. The x coordinate of the sum is $B_1\cos2\pi\omega_0t$ and the y coordinate of the sum is $B_1\sin2\pi\omega_0t$. This is the equation of circular motion. Therefore, the net transverse magnetization of the two coils will be of magnitude B_1 and will rotate in a circle at frequency ω_0. This is precisely how the rotating B_1 field described above is generated. Such a field is usually referred to as being circularly polarized. Similarly, an RF pulse produced by such a rotating field is usually referred to as a circularly polarized RF pulse.

Thus we see that to produce a circularly polarized RF pulse requires two coils oriented at 90° to one another. This is the most efficient means of converting longitudinal magnetization into transverse magnetization. If only one of the coils is used, it will still convert longitudinal magnetization into transverse magnetization, but at a cost of greater energy requirements. The use of a single coil to produce the RF pulse is referred to as a linearly polarized RF pulse. It is also important to note that a circularly polarized RF pulse gives a more homogeneous excitation than a linearly polarized RF pulse.

6 Relaxation Times and Mechanisms

1 IMAGE WEIGHTING

Before discussing the molecular basis of relaxation, the meanings of the terms T1 and T2 relaxation times will be reviewed. Suppose a sample of protons is placed in a magnetic field of strength B_0 aligned along the z axis. At equilibrium, the sample will acquire a net magnetization along the direction of the B_0 field (i.e., along the z axis) because there is a slight excess of protons aligned with the magnetic field. This magnetization is referred to as longitudinal magnetization (M_z). Magnetization perpendicular to this direction (i.e., in the xy plane) is referred to as transverse magnetization (M_{xy}). At equilibrium, the net transverse magnetization of the sample of protons will be zero.

Following a 90° RF pulse, M_z is completely converted into M_{xy}. Since the M_{xy} magnetization is not oriented along the B_0 field, it will precess around the axis of the B_0 field. This rotating magnetization is the origin of the MR signal. However, once the 90° RF pulse is turned off, the system returns to equilibrium: The transverse magnetization decays to zero and the longitudinal magnetization recovers to its initial value prior to the 90° pulse.

Recovery of longitudinal magnetization is referred to as T1 relaxation. This recovery can be described mathematically: denote by $M_z(t)$ the longitudinal magnetization at time t (the subscript z is used because the longitudinal magnetization is along the z axis). Let t = 0 be the time immediately following application of the 90° pulse and let M_z be the value of the longitudinal magnetization just prior to the 90° pulse. It can be shown mathematically and experimentally that recovery of longitudinal magnetization occurs in an exponential fashion such that

$$M_z(t) = M_z[1 - e^{-t/T1}]$$

where e is the base of the natural logarithms (e is approximately 2.71828). Therefore, after a time interval equal to the T1 value, the longitudinal magnetization will have recovered to (1 − 1/e), or 63%, of its equilibrium value. A graph of $M_z(t)$ versus time is shown in Figure 6-1.

Decay of transverse magnetization is referred to as T2 relaxation. This experimentally observed decay can be described mathematically. Denote by $M_{xy}(t)$ the transverse magnetization at time t (the subscript xy is used because the transverse magnetization is within the xy plane). Let t = 0 be the time immediately following application of the 90° pulse. Then, since immediately following the 90° pulse the

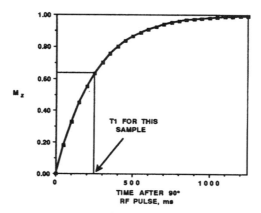

FIGURE 6-1. The recovery of M_z after a 90° RF pulse that has caused M_z to go to zero. T1 is defined as the time for M_z to recover to 63% of its initial value.

initial longitudinal magnetization is completely converted into transverse magnetization $M_{xy}(0) = M_z$. It can be shown mathematically that the decay of transverse magnetization occurs in an exponential fashion such that

$$M_{xy}(t) = M_z[e^{-t/T2}]$$

A graph of $M_{xy}(t)$ versus time is shown in Figure 6-2.

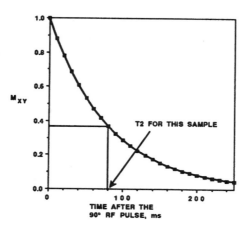

FIGURE 6-2. The decay of M_{xy} after a 90° RF pulse that has caused M_z to be converted to M_{xy}. T2 is defined as the time for M_{xy} to decay to 37% of its initial value.

As noted previously, the magnetic field of clinical imaging systems cannot be made perfectly homogeneous. Following an excitation pulse, the individual protons precess relatively in phase around the B_0 field. The effect of even small differences in the local magnetic field is to cause the precessing protons to get out of phase (referred to as "dephasing"). As a result of this dephasing, the decay of transverse magnetization will actually occur at a faster rate than predicted by the T2 value of body tissues alone. The "net T2 value" due to the inherent tissue T2 and the effect of local field inhomogeneities is usually denoted as T2*. As will be discussed later, the 180° refocusing pulse used with spin echo sequences eliminates the dephasing due to field inhomogeneities and allows true T2 tissue contrast to develop. On the other hand, gradient echo sequences, which do not use a 180° refocusing pulse, will generate images with T2* contrast.

In MRI, many excitation pulses (most commonly 90° pulses) are applied sequentially, with signal measurements performed following each pulse. The time between excitation pulses is denoted by TR. In some imaging sequences, a short series of excitation pulses are applied at TR intervals before the imaging sequence in order to achieve a steady state. The degree of recovery of longitudinal magnetization in each portion of a patient will vary depending upon the local tissue T1 value. However, once a steady state is reached, each portion of a sample will recover the same amount of longitudinal magnetization between excitation pulses. At the time of the next excitation pulse, the recovered longitudinal magnetization will be converted into transverse magnetization. The MR signal is then generated by the precessing transverse magnetization. The signal is measured at time TE following the 90° excitation. The decay of the signal over the time TE is then determined by the T2 (or T2*) value of each portion of the sample.

The recovery of longitudinal magnetization is directly proportional to $M_z[1 - e^{-TR/T1}]$. Note that t has been replaced by TR, the time available for recovery of longitudinal magnetization between successive excitations. The actual amount of longitudinal magnetization present in a small volume of the sample (volume element, or "voxel") is proportional to

$$N(H) \times M_z[1 - e^{-TR/T1}]$$

where N(H) is the density of protons within the voxel. This is the amount of longitudinal magnetization actually available for conversion into transverse magnetization by the 90° pulse. Once converted into transverse magnetization, this magnetization will decay by the factor $[e^{-TE/T2}]$. Note that in this factor, t has been replaced by TE, the time over which the transverse magnetization decays prior to signal measurement. The total MR signal is therefore proportional to

$$N(H) \times M_z[1 - e^{-TR/T1}] \times [e^{-TE/T2}]$$

This equation shows that all MR images, regardless of the parameters chosen, will have signal intensity dependent upon T1, T2, and proton density. However, depending upon the choice of TR and TE, one parameter can be made to dominate the signal intensity characteristics. Hence the term "weighted" is used.

At the time of each 90° pulse, the net longitudinal magnetization becomes zero. During the TR interval, longitudinal magnetization will recover to a degree dependent upon the T1 relaxation time. For tissues with a short T1 (such as lipid), there is more rapid recovery during each TR interval. For tissues with a long T1 (those with a high water content), there is little recovery of longitudinal magnetization when the TR interval is short. This differential recovery of longitudinal magnetization among tissues is a function of their T1 values. When long TR intervals are used almost all tissues undergo complete recovery of longitudinal magnetization (i.e., $[1 - e^{-TR/T1}]$ approaches 1 as TR >> T1 for all tissues). Thus, to eliminate T1 contrast, long TR intervals are used.

The other major factor that determines tissue contrast is echo time (TE). This is the time at which the signal is measured after the 90° pulse. Immediately after a 90° pulse the net transverse magnetization, M_{xy}, is at its maximum. The rate at which the transverse magnetization decays is dependent on T2 (or T2*). The greater the T2 value the longer the transverse magnetization persists. Therefore, in order to develop T2 contrast, the echo time is chosen to be relatively long, so that tissues with short T2 will have lost a significant amount of transverse magnetization and others will have retained a significant amount at the echo time, TE. In order to eliminate (or reduce) T2 contrast, a relatively short echo time is used (i.e., $e^{-TE/T2}$ approaches 1 as TE << T2 for all tissues). Then, no tissue will undergo a significant loss of transverse magnetization over the TE time.

Therefore, a T1-weighted sequence uses a short TR (to develop T1 contrast) and a short TE (to eliminate T2 contrast). At 1.5T, a typical T1-weighted sequence will use TR = 400–600 ms and TE = 10–20 ms. A T2-weighted sequence uses a long TR (to eliminate T1 contrast) and a long TE (to develop T2 contrast). A typical T2-weighted sequence will use TR = 1800–2500 ms and TE = 80–100 ms. By using a long TR to eliminate T1 contrast and a short TE to eliminate T2 contrast, a proton density–weighted image is obtained (e.g., TR = 1800–2500 ms, TE = 10–20 ms).

2   MOLECULAR BASIS OF RELAXATION

As previously discussed, when placed in an external magnetic field, individual protons will assume one of two possible orientations. Let Pr_w and Pr_a denote protons aligned with and against the B_0 field. Since alignment with the (B_0) field is energetically more favorable, the transition from Pr_a to Pr_w is more favorable.

The transition between alignment states is exactly analogous to the chemical equilibrium $Pr_w \rightleftharpoons Pr_a$. The rate of the forward reaction is equal to $C_f[Pr_w]$ and the rate of the reverse reaction is equal to $C_r[Pr_a]$, for some constants C_f and C_r where the term in brackets denotes concentration. Since the reverse reaction is more likely, $C_r > C_f$.

At equilibrium, the forward and reverse reaction rates must be equal. That is, at equilibrium, $C_f[Pr_w] = C_r[Pr_a]$, which is equivalent to $[Pr_w] = (C_r/C_f)[Pr_a]$. Since $C_r > C_f$, $(C_r/C_f) > 1$. Therefore, at equilibrium $[Pr_w] > [Pr_a]$. Thus, there will be a net excess of protons aligned with the B_0 field at equilibrium. The rate at which equilibrium is achieved is dependent upon the constants C_r and C_f. **The greater these constants, the faster equilibrium is achieved**. The equilibrium between alignment states is synonymous with T1 relaxation.

In addition to their alignment with respect to B_0, the individual protons will themselves precess around the axis of the B_0 field. Suppose B_0 is along the z axis.

The rate of rotation is given by $\omega_0 = \gamma B_0$. Consider an individual proton aligned with the B_0 field. In a frame of reference rotating at the rate ω_0 around the z axis, the proton will be fixed. Suppose we apply a weak magnetic field (B_1), which rotates around the z axis (in the xy plane) at the frequency ω_0. Since the proton possesses intrinsic spin, it will want to rotate around the B_1 field. If it were free to rotate, it would rotate toward an orientation against the external field. However, the proton is constrained to be oriented either with or against the B_0 field.

In this circumstance, the proton will be induced to undergo a transition from being aligned with the B_0 field to being aligned against the B_0 field. In an identical manner, if the proton is initially aligned against the B_0 field, the effect of the rotating B_1 field would be to induce a transition from being aligned against the B_0 field to being aligned with the B_0 field. This is strictly a quantum mechanical effect.

Therefore, the effect of the weak rotating magnetic field on an individual proton is to induce a **transition** from one alignment state to another. It is important to note that it will induce transitions in both directions. This is exactly analogous to a catalyst for a chemical reaction. A catalyst serves to increase the rate of both the forward and reverse reactions and therefore increase the rate constants C_f and C_r. This results in an increase in the rate at which equilibrium is achieved. That is, the rotating field will cause T1 relaxation.

It is important to note that only a rotating magnetic field within the xy plane (or having a component within the xy plane) will induce such transitions. How does this relate to the T1 relaxation of water molecules? A water molecule consists of two hydrogen atoms attached to an oxygen atom. Suppose a solution of water molecules is placed in an external magnetic field of strength B_0. The intrinsic magnetic field of the two hydrogen atoms can be aligned either with or against the B_0 field at all times. The water molecules themselves are free to rotate and translate in space. Even as the water molecules rotate and translate in solution, the magnetic field of the individual hydrogen atoms remains aligned either with or against the external field.

As water molecules rotate, the magnetic field associated with the protons they contain also rotates (Figure 6-3). The rotational motion of the water molecules therefore has associated with it an oscillating magnetic field. If the rotation of a water molecule happens to be at the resonance frequency ω_0, then the rotating magnetic field will induce transitions between the alignment states of nearby protons. The nearby protons can be on the same water molecule or on adjacent water molecules. This is precisely the mechanism of T1 relaxation. Since this effect is caused by the interaction of the magnetic field of one proton with another proton, it is usually referred to as a proton–proton interaction (or dipole–dipole interaction).

It is important to note that the strength of the dipole–dipole interaction is inversely proportional to the sixth power of the distance between the interacting dipoles. Therefore, in order to have an effective dipole–dipole interaction, the two dipoles must be able to approach one another very closely.

Only those water molecules (or, if present in solution, other atoms or molecules that possess a dipole moment) rotating at the resonance frequency of the protons (and with their rotational motion having a component within the xy plane) are

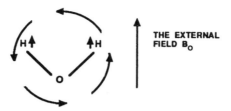

FIGURE 6-3. A water molecule in a magnetic field will have its two protons aligned with or against the external field, B_o. Here, they are shown aligned with B_o. When the molecule as a whole rotates, it carries the proton magnetic moments along.

effective in causing this relaxation. If the water molecules within a solution are free to rotate and move in all directions, there will always be some protons rotating at the resonance frequency with a component in the xy plane. In fact, the frequency of rotation as well as the orientation of the rotation of an individual water molecule will rapidly change over time. Since there is no preferred orientation of the molecules in solution, all possible orientations will be equally likely. This is not true in solids or other structured materials, which will be discussed in more detail later.

Due to variations in thermal energy of individual water molecules, the rate of rotation of individual water molecules will vary. In fact, the distribution of rotation rates will be a Boltzmann type distribution (discussed in Chapter 1), which is dependent upon temperature. That is, at any instant of time within a solution of water molecules, there will be a fixed proportion of water molecules rotating at a given frequency. The frequency of rotation of an individual water molecule may change from one instant to another, but the proportion of water molecules with a given frequency of rotation will remain constant over time. The actual distribution of rotational frequencies will depend upon the temperature.

In pure water at 37°C, the average frequency of rotation of water molecules is much greater than the proton resonance frequency of even the strongest magnetic fields used for MRI. Therefore, at any instant of time, there are relatively few molecules rotating at the resonance frequency. This is why pure water has a very long T1 relaxation time (approximately 3.6 s). Protein molecules, being much larger than water molecules, have an average rotational frequency that is significantly slower than water molecules. In fact, it is much closer to the resonance frequency of the water protons. In water solution, protein molecules can form hydrogen bonds with water protons. This interaction disturbs the molecular motion (i.e., the rotational motion), so that the water molecules rotate more slowly and therefore closer to resonance frequencies of imaging magnets. Thus, protein solutions have a shorter T1 than pure water.

What about the protons in lipid molecules? Most lipids within the human body are contained in triglycerides. These molecules are relatively large and rotate and translate at an average rate much slower than water molecules. In fact, their average rate of rotation will be much closer to the resonance frequency. Therefore, the dipole–dipole interactions in lipids will be significantly greater than that in water. It is for this reason that lipids (in a liquid or semiliquid state) have a very short T1 compared with water. In addition to the rotation of the lipid molecules themselves, their will also be rotation of the $-CH_2$ and $-CH_3$ groups around the carbon–carbon single bonds. This rotational motion will also cause T1 relaxation.

Although not readily apparent, the same dipole–dipole interaction that causes T1 relaxation will also cause T2 relaxation. Immediately following an RF excitation pulse, transverse magnetization is created. While the transverse magnetization persists, the individual protons will rotate around the B_0 field in phase. Independent of the precessional motion, the magnetic field associated with each proton due to its spin will be in one of the two allowable alignment states.

Suppose two protons (denoted by P_1 and P_2) are rotating in phase immediately following an RF pulse. In addition, suppose one of these protons (say, P_1) is induced to change its alignment state by a dipole–dipole interaction with a proton on a nearby rotating water molecule (denoted by W). Even after the change of alignment state, proton P_1 will continue to rotate around the axis of the B_0 field. What happens to the phase of P_1? The phase of P_1 will depend upon the phase of W. But the phase of W is random. Therefore, following the transition, P_1 and P_2 may no longer be in phase. Thus, the transition (due to the dipole–dipole interaction) results in dephasing of the protons P_1 and P_2. This is precisely T2 relaxation. Therefore, transitions induced by a dipole–dipole interaction result in both T1 and T2 relaxation. In fact, the dipole–dipole interaction will affect the T1 and T2 relaxation rates to the same degree. However, this is not the primary mechanism of T2 relaxation.

In solution, the rotational motion of water molecules will be distributed over a range of frequencies dependent upon the temperature. Most water molecules will be rotating very rapidly (in fact, greatly exceeding the resonance frequency of 63.87 MHz at 1.5 T). However, some water molecules will be rotating relatively slowly. These water molecules will be relatively fixed in orientation.

What happens when water molecules are relatively fixed in orientation and position in space? In the vicinity of such water molecules, the local magnetic field will be slightly different from B_0. Therefore, protons in the vicinity of such fixed water molecules will precess at a frequency slightly different from 63.87 MHz. This results in dephasing of transverse magnetization. Hence, the effect of the fixed water molecules is to cause T2 relaxation — the decay of M_{xy}.

This effect of the relatively fixed water molecules is separate from the dipole–dipole interaction. This effect is very small in pure water because there are very few water molecules that are relatively fixed. Thus, pure water has a very long T2 relaxation time (about 3.6 s). However, in proteinaceous solutions, water molecules rotate more slowly. Therefore, there will be a relatively large number of fixed water molecules. This causes significant T2 shortening in proteinaceous solutions. In fact, this effect is most pronounced in solids, where there is little rotation of proteins or water molecules.

It is the presence of these relatively fixed water molecules in most biologic tissues that causes biologic tissues to have a T2 that is significantly shorter than that of pure water. This effect also results in an interesting phenomenon in collagenous tissues, which will be discussed later.

To summarize,

1. The rotational motion of molecules in solution results in both T1 and T2 relaxation through the dipole–dipole interaction. The closer the frequency of the rotational motion to the resonance frequency of the protons, the more effective is the dipole–dipole interaction.
2. Those water molecules that are relatively fixed (in orientation and position) result in a field heterogeneity that causes selective T2 relaxation (by selective is meant T2 but not T1 relaxation). This effect is independent from the dipole–dipole interaction. In this context, relatively fixed means a rotational frequency significantly less than the typical proton resonance frequencies of MRI magnets. Thus, even if the rotational frequency is as low as 1 MHz (which is **one million** cycles per second), this is still slow compared with 63 million cycles per second.

3   PARAMAGNETIC RELAXATION EFFECTS

How do paramagnetic species (including contrast agents) affect MR signal characteristics? Many metals exist in water solutions as charged ions. Gadolinium ions (Gd^{3+}) contain a large number of unpaired electrons (seven in the case of Gd^{3+}) that are paramagnetic. Therefore, these species act as strong dipoles. In solution, free Gd^{3+} is not effective at causing relaxation through a dipole–dipole interaction. This is because the Gd atom is very small and therefore has a very rapid rate of rotation (much more rapid than the resonance frequency of protons). However, when attached to a large molecule such as diethylene triamine pentaacetic acid (DTPA), the Gd-DTPA molecule rotates more slowly, at a rate much closer (on average) to the resonance frequency of water protons. This is why Gd-DTPA is an effective relaxation agent.

For this same reason, methemoglobin is an effective relaxation agent. Methemoglobin is a large molecule (with a slow rate of rotation) that contains Fe^{3+}. Fe^{3+} is strongly paramagnetic because it contains five unpaired electrons. Why, then, is deoxyhemoglobin (which is a large molecule that is strongly paramagnetic because it contains Fe^{2+} with four unpaired electrons) not an effective relaxation agent?

Due to its molecular structure (which is different from methemoglobin), the Fe atom in deoxyhemoglobin is relatively inaccessible to water protons in solution. This means that water protons in solution cannot closely approach the Fe atom in deoxyhemoglobin. Because the water protons cannot closely approach it, the dipole–dipole interaction is exceedingly weak. This results from the fact that the dipole–dipole interaction scales as the sixth power of distance between the interacting species.

However, if deoxyhemoglobin is sequestered within red blood cells, then the field within and near such red blood cells will be greater than that outside of the red blood cells. This creates a local field inhomogeneity, which results in selective T2 relaxation (just as relatively stationary water molecules can result in selective T2 relaxation). Therefore, intracellular (i.e., in red blood cells) deoxyhemoglobin will cause selective T2 relaxation. Likewise, intracellular methemoglobin will cause selective T2 relaxation in addition to both T1 and T2 relaxation through the dipole–dipole interaction.

Paramagnetic agents such as Gd-DTPA cause both T1 and T2 relaxation through the dipole–dipole interaction. Why, then, do these agents seem to selectively affect the contrast of T1-weighted images (and not T2-weighted images)? This results from the fact that the dipole–dipole interaction equally affects the relaxation *rates* (not the relaxation times).

The relaxation rate is the reciprocal of the relaxation time (i.e., R1 = 1/T1 and R2 = 1/T2). For virtually all tissues, T1 >> T2. Therefore, for virtually all tissues, R2 >> R1. As an example, suppose a tissue has R1 = 10 units and R2 = 100 units, using some arbitrary scale. In addition, suppose a paramagnetic agent, such as Gd-DTPA, increases both the R1 and R2 relaxation rates by 10. This causes doubling of the T1 relaxation rate (form 10 to 20) but only a 10% increase in the T2 relaxation rate (from 100 to 110). The actual effect is of course dependent upon the concentration of the Gd-DTPA. At the concentrations used for clinical imaging, Gd-DTPA essentially causes only significant T1 relaxation within body tissues.

Some interesting effects of Gd-DTPA may be observed in the bladder. Images obtained several minutes following intravenous administration of Gd-DTPA show effects relating to both T1 and T2 relaxation. This is manifest as three distinct regions of signal intensity within the urine-filled bladder. Due to differential layering of the Gd-DTPA molecules, there will be a concentration gradient from the most dependent to the least dependent portions of the bladder.

In the most dependent portion of the bladder, the concentration of Gd-DTPA will be high and result in significant T1 and T2 relaxation. Due to the significant T2 relaxation (i.e., decrease of T2), this portion of the bladder will have a signal void (i.e., appear black) even on T1-weighted images. This results from the fact that if the T2 relaxation time is short enough, there will be so much dephasing even at short echo times that no measurable signal will be left.

In the central part of the bladder, the Gd-DTPA concentration is such that there is significant T1 relaxation but little T2 relaxation. This portion of the bladder will have a very high signal (i.e., appear white) on T1-weighted images. In the least dependent portion of the bladder, the Gd-DTPA concentration is such that there is not significant T1 or T2 relaxation. This portion of the bladder will have the signal intensity of normal urine, which is relatively gray on T1-weighted images.

One might expect that these variations of signal intensity within the bladder would be gradual. However, if one plots the variation of signal intensity (of water containing Gd-DTPA) versus the concentration of Gd-DTPA, the resulting curve has a sharp peak. The signal intensity has a maximum value at some concentration C, and the signal intensity then drops off very rapidly (due to T2 effects) for concentrations greater than or less than C.

4 MAGNETIZATION TRANSFER EFFECTS

Suppose a solution of water molecules is placed in a perfectly homogeneous magnetic field of strength B_0. Even though the field is perfectly homogeneous, the protons within the sample will not precess at exactly the same frequency. This results from interactions between adjacent water molecules. Recall that the water molecules within a solution will rotate and translate. The rotational frequencies will vary according to a Boltzmann distribution. That is, some water molecules will rotate more rapidly than others. The distribution of rotational frequencies will be around a mean frequency. The mean frequency is determined by the temperature (as well as the presence of other molecules, such as protein molecules, which can interact with [or disturb] the rotation of the water molecules).

Water molecules that rotate slowly (i.e., are relatively fixed in orientation) cause small local field differences within the solution. These local field differences cause water protons to have different resonance frequencies at different locations within the solution. If the mean frequency of rotation of the water molecules is relatively high, compared with the resonance frequency of the water protons, then there will be very few fixed water molecules. In this solution, virtually all water molecules will have the same resonance frequency. Hence, the spectrum of frequencies of such a solution will have a very narrow peak, centered around the mean frequency.

On the other hand, if the mean frequency of rotation of the water molecules is relatively slow compared with the resonance frequency of the water protons, then there will be a large number of fixed water molecules. In this solution, the water molecules will be precessing at many different frequencies. Hence, the spectrum of frequencies of such a solution will have a very broad peak, centered around the mean frequency.

Following an excitation pulse, the transverse magnetization within a sample will precess at a frequency that is directly proportional to the local magnetic field strength. If there is a broad variability in local field strength, there will be more variability in the precessional frequency of the transverse magnetization, producing rapid dephasing of the transverse magnetization. This is precisely T2 relaxation.

In simpler terms, then, solutions with a narrow band of resonance frequencies will have a long T2 relaxation time and solutions with a broad band of resonance frequencies will have a short T2 relaxation time (Figure 6-4).

Consider a dilute solution of protein molecules in water. At any instant of time, most of the water molecules will not be associated with (or influenced by) the protein molecules in solution. These water molecules are usually referred to as bulk water (or free water) molecules. A portion of the water molecules will interact with the protein molecules (via hydrogen bonds) and as a result will have their rotational motion slowed. These water molecules are usually referred to as hydration (or bound) water molecules.

It is important to note that there is a constant exchange between the free water molecules and the hydration water molecules. An equilibrium is quickly established between the two groups. At equilibrium, the number of free water molecules and the number of hydration water molecules will remain fixed. However, individual water molecules still exchange between the two groups.

The free water molecules will have a relatively narrow band of resonance frequencies and will therefore have a relatively long T2 relaxation time. The hydration water molecules will have a relatively broad NMR peak and will therefore have a relatively short T2 relaxation time (Figure 6-4). At 1.5 T, both groups of water molecules will have resonance frequency centered around 63.87 MHz. Denote the

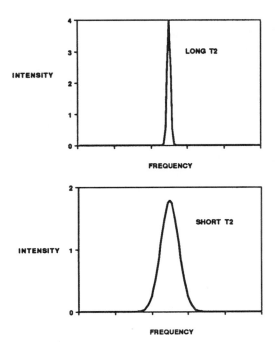

FIGURE 6-4. Solutions with a narrow band of resonance frequencies (top) will have a long T2, but solutions with a wide band of resonance frequencies (bottom) will have a short T2.

range (or bandwidth) of resonance frequencies in the free water fraction as ΔB_F. Denote the range of resonance frequencies in the hydration water fraction as ΔB_H. Then ΔB_H greatly exceeds ΔB_F.

The free water protons will have resonance frequencies in the range from 63.87 MHz $- \Delta B_F$ to 63.87 MHz $+ \Delta B_F$. The hydration water protons will have resonance frequencies in the range from 63.87 MHz $- \Delta B_H$ to 63.87 MHz $+ \Delta B_H$.

Suppose such a solution is exposed to an RF excitation pulse centered at 63.87 MHz and with bandwidth ΔB, such that $\Delta B > \Delta B_H$. This will result in excitation of both the free and hydration water molecules. This is how a standard excitation pulse is applied.

Suppose such a solution is exposed to an RF excitation pulse centered at 63.87 MHz $\pm \Delta B$, where $\Delta B_F < \Delta B < \Delta B_H$. Such a pulse is referred to as an off-resonance pulse because it is not centered at 63.87 MHz. None of the free water protons will have resonance frequencies in this range and therefore the free water protons will not be excited. However, a large number of the hydration water protons will have resonance frequencies in this range and will therefore be excited. Therefore, the effect of the off-resonance excitation pulse is to selectively excite the hydration water protons.

Suppose a 90° off-resonance excitation pulse is applied to a water solution of protein molecules. The hydration water molecules will undergo complete loss of longitudinal magnetization associated with creation of transverse magnetization. Due to the very short T2 of hydration water molecules, the transverse magnetization will undergo almost immediate decay. Therefore, the net effect of the off-resonance pulse is to cause loss of longitudinal magnetization of the hydration water protons.

Therefore, following the off-resonance excitation pulse, there will be an equal number of hydration water protons aligned with or opposite the external magnetic field. Since the free water protons were unaffected by the off-resonance pulse, there will still be a net excess of free water protons aligned with the external field. That is, the group of hydration water protons will have zero net longitudinal magnetization and the group of free water protons will have nonzero net longitudinal magnetization along the direction of the external field.

However, the hydration water protons can exchange with free water protons (and vice versa). As this occurs, there will be a net loss of longitudinal magnetization in the group of free water protons and a corresponding net gain of longitudinal magnetization in the group of hydration water protons. This is equivalent to a net transfer of longitudinal magnetization from the free water protons to the hydration water protons. Hence the name **magnetization transfer**.

Due to the very short T2 of hydration water protons, the signal from the solution of water and protein molecules is entirely determined by the free water protons. Now, suppose an imaging sequence is performed following the application of an off-resonance excitation pulse. The loss of longitudinal magnetization of the free water protons resulting from magnetization transfer will cause signal loss.

The degree of signal loss from magnetization transfer effects will be directly proportional to the ratio of the number of hydration water molecules to free water molecules. Magnetization transfer effects will therefore be zero for pure water, which contains only free water molecules. Most biologic tissues will have varying degrees of hydration water molecules and will therefore have varying degrees of magnetization transfer effects. This provides another means of developing contrast in MRI separate from T1 and T2 effects.

5   MAGIC ANGLE PHENOMENON

When the rotational motion of water molecules is very slow compared with the resonance frequency of the water protons, there is selective T2 shortening. Therefore, if a tissue contains water molecules that are highly structured (i.e., have restricted motion), it will have a very short T2 relaxation time. Such tissues will usually appear dark on all pulse sequences, even T1- and proton density–weighted images. This results from the fact that for such tissues, the term $e^{-TE/T2}$ will be close to zero and hence will dominate the signal intensity of the tissue.

Ice is an example of highly structured water molecules. The T2 value of ice is so short that it will have very low signal intensity on all pulse sequences. This results from the fact that no matter how short the TE that is chosen, there will be complete dephasing of the signal by the time of signal measurement.

Another example of a tissue that consists of highly structured water molecules is tendon. Tendon consists largely of collagen. Even when a tendon is injured and becomes edematous, its T2 relaxation time remains relatively short. Therefore, edematous tendon will still have very low signal intensity on T2-weighted images.

However, edematous tendon can have increased signal intensity on T1- and proton density–weighted images. This paradoxical behavior results from the fact that edema increases the T2 relaxation time sufficiently such that some signal will be seen if a very short TE is used. However, even in the presence of edema, the T2 relaxation time is still so short that there is no signal on long TE images. If, however, the collagen fibrils are disrupted such that a small pocket of fluid is present within the substance of the tendon, then it will appear as fluid-like signal intensity on T2-weighted images.

Due to its highly organized structure, all the collagen fibrils that make up a tendon will be oriented in nearly the same direction. Most of the water molecules in a tendon will be hydration water and will strongly interact with the molecules of collagen microfibrils. This will cause the water molecules to become oriented along the direction of the microfibrils. Hence, there will be a preferred direction of orientation of the water molecules.

Now, the decrease in T2 relaxation of hydration water protons is due to fixed local field changes induced by adjacent hydration water protons. However, only alterations of the field strength along the z direction will cause T2 shortening. This is because the precessional frequency of the water protons (around the axis of the external field) is solely determined by the local field strength along the direction of the external field. For example, if the local field is changed along the x or y directions, this will not alter the precessional frequency around the z axis.

One water proton interacts with an adjacent water proton through its associated magnetic field. The magnetic field of a water proton is approximately that of a dipole. Each dipole must be oriented either with or opposed to the external magnetic field. Only that component of the dipole field oriented along the z direction will cause a local change in precessional frequency. It can be shown that the field of a dipole located at the origin of a Cartesian coordinate system will have a z component of magnitude $(3\cos^2\Theta - 1)/r^3$ at a point located a distance r from the origin and oriented at an angle Θ with respect to the z axis.

Suppose a tendon (and hence its microfibrils) is oriented at an angle Θ with respect to the z axis. Consider two adjacent hydration water molecules. They will be oriented along the axis of the tendon. Hence, if a line is drawn between the two adjacent hydration water molecules, this line will be oriented at an angle Θ with respect to the z axis. Hence, the z field experienced by one hydration water proton due to an adjacent hydration water proton will be proportional to $(3\cos^2\Theta - 1)/r^3$. If Θ is such that $(3\cos^2\Theta - 1) = 0$, then the interaction between adjacent hydration water protons will be negligible. In this circumstance, there will be no T2 shortening, and therefore no signal loss.

Therefore, when a tendon is oriented at an angle Θ with respect to the external magnetic field such that $(3\cos^2\Theta - 1) = 0$, there will not be significant T2 shortening. The tendon will therefore have increased signal and will usually appear gray on T1- and proton density–weighted images. Now, $(3\cos^2\Theta - 1) = 0$ when Θ is approximately **54.7°**. This is the so called **magic angle**. It is important to note this effect because it can result in increased signal within a tendon, which should not be confused with a pathologic abnormality.

7 The Imaging Process

In the preceding chapter, it was shown how a signal can be generated from a collection of protons placed within an external magnetic field and exposed to an RF pulse. However, if all protons within a collection experience the same magnetic field strength, they will all produce a signal at an identical frequency, and they will all be excited by a given RF pulse. In order to generate a useful image, however, selective portions (i.e., sections) of a patient must be excited, and the signal emitted from the patient must be spatially encoded. These are accomplished in several independent steps.

If no other external magnetic field other than the B_0 field is applied, then all portions of a collection of protons placed within the B_0 field will experience equal field strength. Under these circumstances all protons in the collection will precess at the same frequency. Thus, an RF pulse at the resonance frequency will excite the entire collection of protons. In addition, transverse magnetization created by an RF pulse will precess at an identical frequency in all portions of the collection. Therefore, the signal will have the same frequency for all portions of the collection.

In order to distinguish different parts of a collection of protons, the magnetic field strength must be made to vary slightly from point to point. This is achieved by applying gradient fields. These gradient fields are transient small magnetic fields superimposed on the main B_0 field. The gradient fields are turned on only temporarily during application of an RF pulse and during spatial encoding.

If a small gradient field is applied along a specified direction, the precessional frequencies of the protons will vary from point to point. It is important to note that by gradient is meant a change in the strength of the magnetic field along a chosen axis. The direction of the gradient field (as well as the B_0 field) is always along the z axis, but the change in field strength can be made to vary as a function of the x, y, or z coordinate. For example, when a gradient is applied along the x axis, the strength of magnetic field will vary as a function of position along the x axis, but the net magnetic field itself will still be oriented along the z axis. There is no net field component along the x axis when an x gradient is applied.

The strength of the gradients typically used in MRI are very small (0.1 to 1.0 G/cm) compared with the strength of the main field. Therefore, when gradients are applied, they induce only very small changes in the magnetic field strength from point to point (as compared with the main field strength). As a result, when a gradient is applied, the difference in precessional frequency from point to point is also very small.

When magnetic field gradients are applied to a collection of protons, the resonance frequency will be different for different portions of the collection. Therefore, in order to selectively excite a portion of the collection, RF pulses will actually contain a narrow band (or range) of frequencies. The center of this band is usually referred to as the center frequency (or carrier frequency) and the range of frequencies around this center frequency is referred to as the bandwidth of the RF pulse. For example, an RF pulse with a center frequency of 63.87 MHz and a bandwidth of ±16 kHz will contain all frequencies from (63.87 MHz − 16 kHz) to (63.87 MHz + 16 kHz).

Suppose a gradient is applied along the z axis such that the protons within a 1.0-cm thick axial section of tissue will be precessing in a known narrow band of frequencies. If the band of frequencies of an RF pulse exactly matches this band of frequencies, then only those protons within that axial section will be excited. Protons outside of this section will be precessing at frequencies greater or less than those contained in the applied pulse. Remember, protons will be excited only when the frequency of the RF pulse matches the resonance frequency.

This gradient is referred to as the **section select** (or **slice select**) **gradient** because it selectively excites only a specified thin section of tissue. This gradient is on only during the excitation process. Once selective excitation is completed, the gradient is turned off and all of the protons in the sample (including the excited section) will once again precess at the same frequency. This means that the transverse magnetization created in the excited section will also emit signal at the same frequency everywhere in the excited section once the gradient is turned off.

In a similar manner, by applying gradients along the y or x direction, coronal or sagittal sections, respectively, can be selectively excited. If nothing else were done, however, whatever plane of section is selectively excited, the received signal would still represent a composite signal from all of the protons within the excited section.

It now remains to spatially encode the signal from the excited section so that a useful image can be obtained. This is accomplished by two separate processes. Suppose we are dealing with an axial section so that the section select gradient is applied along the z axis as previously described. Once a section is selectively excited, we still have to spatially encode the received signal along the x and y axes. Prior to the signal measurement process a small gradient can be applied along the y axis. While this gradient is on, the precessional frequency of the transverse magnetization within the excited section will vary as a function of position along the y axis.

Once this gradient is turned off, all portions of the sample will again experience the same field strength and the transverse magnetization will then precess at the same frequency in all portions of the excited section. However, while the gradient is on, transverse magnetization in some portions of the excited section will precess more rapidly than in others. The temporary difference in precessional frequencies will change the phase of the rotating transverse magnetization as a function of position along the y axis (Figure 7-1). This effect will persist even when the y gradient is no longer on. That is, even after the y gradient is turned off and all transverse magnetization in the excited section precesses at the same frequency, the phase differences will persist as a function of y. This gradient is referred to as the **phase-encoding gradient**.

What is the phase of a signal? When a signal (or function) is periodic in time (or space), this means that it repeats itself. Trigonometric functions, such as a sine wave, are good examples of periodic functions. The function $\sin\vartheta$ repeats every

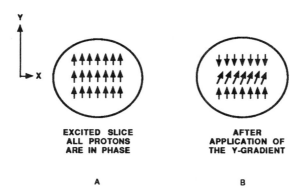

FIGURE 7-1. (A) After selective excitation, all protons in the section are precessing in phase in the xy plane. (B) After the y gradient is applied along the section, the protons acquire a phase that is a function of the strength of the gradient and position along the y axis.

360°. The function $\sin(\Theta + 90°)$ also repeats every 360°. When plotted as a function of Θ, the graphs of these two functions will have an identical appearance except that they are shifted along the Θ axis by 90° (Figure 7-2). These functions are said to have a phase difference of 90°. The function $\sin(\Theta + 90°)$ is said to have a phase of positive 90° with respect to the function $\sin \Theta$. Instead of describing the phase change in terms of degrees, it is commonly expressed in terms of numbers of cycles. For example, since 360° equals one full cycle, a phase change of 90° corresponds to a difference of one-quarter of a cycle.

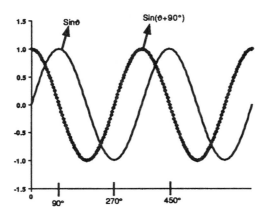

FIGURE 7-2. The periodic trigonometric sine function, plotted as a function of angle from 0 to 360°. One curve is shifted in phase by 90°, but the two curves are otherwise identical.

Phase is a relative value and is always defined with respect to some (arbitrary) reference. In the above case, the reference is the function $\sin \Theta$. We could just as easily have used $\sin(\Theta + 90°)$ as the reference, in which case we would say that the function $\sin (\Theta)$ has a phase of negative 90° with respect to the function $\sin(\Theta + 90°)$.

It is easy to see that a phase change of negative 90° is equivalent to a phase change of positive 270°. Phase changes ($\Delta\phi$) are therefore usually defined such that $-180° \leq \Delta\phi \leq +180°$. This is because a phase change of $180° + \Delta\phi$ is equivalent to a phase change of $-(180° - \Delta\phi)$.

Finally, during the process of signal measurement, a gradient can be applied along the x axis such that the precessional frequencies of transverse magnetization within the excited section will vary depending upon position along the x axis. This gradient is referred to as the **read** or **frequency-encoding gradient**. It is important to note that this is the only gradient that is on during the actual signal measurement. As a result of this gradient, the MR signal is equal to the sum of many signals at different frequencies. Only the overall (or total) signal can be measured. The bandwidth of the signal is determined by the bandwidth of the frequency-encoding gradient.

The time interval between center of application of the RF pulse and the center of the signal measurement process is denoted by TE (<u>t</u>ime of <u>e</u>cho). The measured signal will therefore consist of a superposition of signals at different frequencies. Each frequency component corresponds to a different position along the x axis. In addition, each frequency component is itself a superposition of signals with different phases. The phase of each component is dependent upon position along the y axis.

The received signal is an analog signal (which is a continuous function of time). The received signal is actually "sampled" (i.e., measured) at multiple discrete points of time (typically a power of 2 such as 256 times) during the signal measurement process. The interval of time between signal samples is referred to as the sampling interval. The total time over which all samples are taken is referred to as the sampling time. In this manner, an analog signal is converted into a digital signal (which is a discrete function of time). The number of samples taken is equal to the size of the image matrix along the frequency direction. This process will be discussed in much greater detail in Chapter 8.

It can be shown mathematically that a discrete Fourier transform can be applied to convert the digital signal into multiple (typically 256) component frequencies. Recall that the total MR signal is actually equal to a sum of many signals at different frequencies due to application of the frequency-encoding gradient. A Fourier transform converts a function of time or position (expressed as signal intensity at a given time or location) into a function of frequency (expressed as signal intensity at a given frequency). In this manner, the Fourier transform determines the signal intensity of each of the component frequencies of the MR signal. Since each frequency corresponds to a different spatial location along the frequency-encoding axis, positional information is regained.

Therefore, after performing a Fourier transform on the received signal, we will have determined the signal intensity of the 256 component frequencies. But each of these 256 frequencies consists of many phase components. The number of phase components equals the size of the image matrix along the phase-encoding direction (typically 128, 192, or 256). The signal intensity of each phase component cannot be measured directly. Only the composite signal at each frequency can be determined. Therefore, if, for example, a 128-phase matrix is used, an individual signal measurement yields 256 different signal intensities, each of which equals the sum of 128 *unknown* phase components. In order to determine these 128 unknown quantities, 128 different equations must be generated (to solve for n unknowns requires n equations).

If we repeat the signal measurement process 128 times, 128 equations are generated for each frequency component. The phase gradient is varied for each measurement in order to generate data that is not redundant. This process is equivalent to sampling the phase data just as we sampled the frequency data in order to be able to perform a Fourier transform. The interval of time between repeated measurements is denoted as the TR (time of repetition).

The need for performing many signal measurements can also be given in terms of the Fourier transform. MR signal measurements are performed in the presence of the frequency-encoding gradient. Following each individual excitation, a single phase-encoding gradient is applied and the signal is sampled in the presence of the frequency-encoding gradient. Denote the n-th phase-encoding gradient by G_n. If the phase matrix size is 128, then n varies from 1 to 128. Each signal sample is obtained at a fixed point in time following application of the frequency-encoding gradient. Denote the m-th such time as t_m. If the frequency matrix is 256, then m varies from 1 to 256. Each signal sample can then be identified by the phase-encoding gradient strength applied prior to signal measurement as well as the time of measurement following turning on of the frequency-encoding gradient. Each signal sample can then be denoted by $S(G_n, t_m)$.

For each value of G_n, there will be 256 different values of S (corresponding to each value of t_m). These values can be Fourier transformed to yield the amplitudes of the different frequency components in each signal due to the frequency-encoding gradient. The only way to keep G_n fixed and vary t_m is to apply a single phase-encoding gradient and measure the signal over time following application of the frequency-encoding gradient. However, each of these frequency components consists of many different phase components.

For each value of t_m, there will be 128 different values of S. These values can be Fourier transformed to yield the amplitudes of the different phase components in each signal due to the phase-encoding gradient. The only way to keep t_m fixed and vary G_n is to repeat the measurement process 128 times each time with a different phase-encoding gradient strength. This is precisely what is done to generate all of the necessary information to spatially encode an MR image.

Up to this point, then, the MRI process consists of the following steps:

- A collection of protons (i.e., a patient) is placed within a strong homogeneous external magnetic field of known strength (B_0).
- A small magnetic field gradient is applied along the x, y, or z axis. For illustrative purposes assume this gradient is applied along the z axis to generate an axial section.
- An RF pulse is applied in a specific frequency range to selectively excite a thin section at a specific location. For most applications, optimal excitation is achieved by using a 90° circularly polarized RF pulse.

- A small gradient is applied along the y axis to induce phase changes as a function of position along the y axis. This is done after the 90° pulse but prior to signal measurement.
- At a specified time (TE) following the 90° pulse, a small gradient is applied along the x axis and the signal is measured in the presence of this gradient.
- This process is repeated as many times as there are phase-encoding steps, each time with a different strength phase-encoding gradient.

For most applications, the time between measurements (the TR) is much greater than TE. This allows many different sections to be excited during the same TR interval, because once the signal is measured from one section there is nothing left to do with that section until the TR interval has expired. Most MR sequences consist of multisection acquisitions. In addition, in order to improve the S/N, not only is the process repeated 128 times for 128 phase-encoding steps, but it can be repeated several times for each phase-encoding step. The number of excitations per phase-encoding step is usually referred to as the number of signal averages (NSA), or number of excitations (NEX).

Therefore, the total imaging time for the MRI sequence as described above is given by

Total imaging time = (TR) × (NSA) × (Number of phase encodings)

The imaging sequence described up to this point leaves out one important facet. Ideally, the main external magnetic field would be of equal magnitude at all points within the magnet. In reality, however, small inhomogeneities always persist. This results in fixed inhomogeneity in the main magnetic field. That is, due to field inhomogeneity, some places within the bore of the magnet will always be at slightly higher (or lower) field strengths than others. These fixed inhomogeneities cause local differences in precessional frequencies.

What is the effect on the MR signal of local inhomogeneities in the main magnetic field? Because the transverse magnetization created by an RF pulse precesses about the axis of the main magnetic field to generate the MR signal, the frequency of this precession (and hence the frequency of the signal) in any small region of a patient being imaged is dependent upon the local field strength.

The signal will be greatest in a small region if all of the transverse magnetization within that region precesses at precisely the same frequency. Otherwise, if there is precession at many different frequencies, the individual signals in even very small regions (such as individual voxels) will rapidly get out of phase and the signal will decay very rapidly. This type of signal loss is said to be due to **dephasing**.

Were it not compensated for, this dephasing would cause significant signal loss in clinical imaging. In order to compensate for fixed inhomogeneities of the main external field, an additional RF pulse is incorporated into each imaging sequence. This additional pulse is actually a 180° pulse that is applied at time TE/2 after each 90° RF pulse. This works as follows:

Transverse magnetization in a region of higher field strength precesses slightly faster than in the weaker areas of the field and therefore acquires a relative positive phase. This can be thought of as some transverse magnetization precessing ahead of other transverse magnetization. Following application of a 180° pulse, this phase relationship is reversed, such that transverse magnetization that had been precessing ahead gets behind. Because the transverse magnetization that is then behind is still in the stronger field (assuming the inhomogeneities are fixed), it will once again catch up (Figure 7-3).

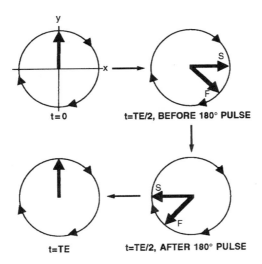

Figure 7-3. At time t = 0, (just after a 90° RF pulse), the net transverse magnetization is shown rotating clockwise around the z axis in the xy plane. All of the protons have been rotated into the xy plane and they start to precess in phase. At time TE/2, just before the 180° RF pulse, the slower proton (S) is oriented along the positive x axis and the faster proton (F) is oriented slightly ahead in a clockwise direction. At time TE/2, just after the 180° pulse, the order of the protons is reversed since the 180° pulse causes both protons to rotate around the y axis. The slower proton (S) now is ahead of the faster proton (F). At time TE, the faster proton will "catch up" to the slower proton so that both will be in phase.

Why does this work? Suppose there is a fixed inhomogeneity in the main field such that transverse magnetization F (for fast) precesses slightly faster than transverse magnetization S (for slow). Immediately following a 90° RF pulse, both will be in phase. Immediately after the 90° pulse, they will both rotate around the z axis. Suppose that at a later time (TE/2), S is oriented along the positive x axis and F is oriented slightly ahead in a clockwise direction.

Suppose the 180° pulse rotates magnetization around the y axis (this means that the B₁ field is oriented along the x axis). S will be rotated 180° to the negative x axis. F will be rotated 180° to a position slightly behind S (with respect to the clockwise direction). Both will continue to rotate clockwise, with F now slightly behind S but with F continuing to rotate at a faster rate. After another interval of time TE/2 (i.e., at time TE after the initial 90° pulse), F will catch up to S and they will be exactly in phase at that instant. With time, however, they will once again get out of phase.

By applying the 180° pulse, the decay in signal that would otherwise occur due to a field inhomogeneity is canceled out at time TE when the signal is measured. In fact, the signal initially decays up to the time of the 180° RF pulse. The signal then transiently increases to a maximal value at time TE at which time signal measurement is performed. The transient increase in signal caused by the 180° pulse is like an **echo**. It is due to the rotation (or **spin**) of the magnetization by the 180° pulse. Hence the term **spin echo** sequence is applied to sequences that use a 180° RF pulse.

What effects do all of the gradients have on the imaging process? For a spin echo pulse sequence, four separate gradients are used: the section select gradient for the 90° pulse, the section select gradient for the 180° pulse, the phase-encoding gradient, and the frequency-encoding gradient.

All gradients will induce phase changes along the direction of the gradient. This is because all gradients induce changes in the frequency of rotation of transverse magnetization. The gradients have no effect on longitudinal magnetization since, by definition, longitudinal magnetization does not rotate. It is desirable for only the phase-encoding gradient to induce phase changes. Any other gradient-induced phase changes will result in signal loss without serving any other useful purpose.

Suppose a gradient is turned on along the z axis such that the magnetic field strength at any point, B(x,y,z), is given by $B(x,y,z) = B_0 + z\Delta B$, where $\Delta B > 0$. Then, while the gradient is on, the field strength will be greater than B_0 for points along the positive z axis and less than B_0 for points along the negative z axis. Suppose the gradient is on for a time interval Δt. If a second gradient is turned on for time Δt such that $B(x,y,z) = B_0 - z\Delta B$, then the phase changes induced by the first gradient will be exactly reversed by the second gradient. The net phase change induced by both gradients will therefore be zero. A gradient structure that induces no net phase change is called a balanced gradient.

Several other important facts must be kept in mind. The gradient described above caused the local field strength to vary as a function of position along the z axis in a linear manner (i.e., the field strength is proportional to z, as opposed to, say, z^2 or z^3). All of the gradients used in MRI are in fact linear gradients. Also, when a gradient is turned on, it cannot be turned on instantaneously. It takes a small but finite amount of time to reach full strength and actually be linear (i.e., "flat-topped") (Figure 7-4). Therefore, when section selective RF excitation pulses are used, they are actually applied at the center of the gradient. That is, the gradient is on for a brief time before, during, and after the pulse is actually applied. It is simplest to picture the RF pulse as being applied at the exact center of the time during which the gradient is on, and 90° rotation (following a 90° RF pulse) to take place at that time.

It is important to remember that a gradient will induce phase changes only in transverse magnetization. Longitudinal magnetization will not be affected because it is not rotating.

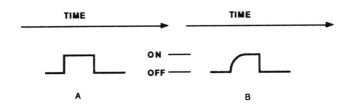

FIGURE 7-4. (A) An ideal gradient, which reaches full strength instantaneously when turned on. (B) A real gradient, which takes some time (known as the gradient rise time) to reach full strength. The rise time must be allowed for when an RF pulse is to be delivered to excite a section.

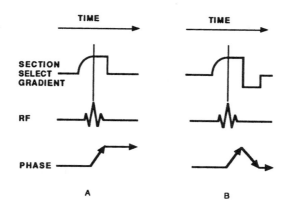

FIGURE 7-5. (A) The 90° RF pulse is applied at the center of the time when the section select gradient is on. Because the gradient remains on after the 90° RF, the protons that have been rotated into the xy plane will develop a phase difference through the slice from back to front. (B) If the section select gradient is reversed and remains on for the same time that it was on after the 90° RF, the phase difference is corrected. The gradient is said to be bilobed. The last lobe is sometimes referred to as the rephasing lobe.

Now return to each of the individual gradients. Prior to the 90° pulse, there is no transverse magnetization. Because the 90° pulse is applied at the center of its section select gradient, it will induce phase changes only during the second half of the gradient. Therefore, in order to compensate for these phase changes, we need only apply a gradient of equal strength and opposite direction for half as long. Therefore, the section select gradient will be bilobed (Figure 7-5). The RF pulse is applied at the center of the first lobe, and the second lobe is of equal magnitude, opposite direction, and half the duration of the first lobe.

The situation with the 180° pulse is somewhat more complicated. Transverse magnetization that is created by the 90° pulse will exist for the entire time that the section select gradient for the 180° pulse is on. The 180° pulse will be applied at the center of the gradient. However, any phase change induced by the first half of the section select gradient for the 180° pulse will actually be reversed by the 180°

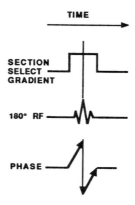

FIGURE 7-6.   During the first half of the time that the section select gradient is on, a phase difference will develop through the section from back to front. The bottom of the figure shows the phase changes at the front of the section, where the gradient is high. The 180° RF pulse reverses this phase difference, so that the gradient must remain on in the same direction during the second half of the section select gradient, to bring the phase difference back to zero.

pulse itself. Therefore, in order to cancel out these phase changes, the second half of the gradient must be of equal magnitude, equal duration, and same direction as the first half (Figure 7-6). In reality, the section select gradient for a 180° pulse is slightly more complex, but this point will be discussed in a later chapter.

The frequency-encoding gradient must be turned on during the signal measurement process. The signal measurement process will be centered around the TE and will take a small but finite amount of time. This means that the read gradient must be on for a short time before and a short time after the TE. It is most convenient for signal measurement purposes for the signal to be maximal (and therefore symmetric) about the TE. For this reason, it is customary to have all phase changes induced by the frequency-encoding gradient to be exactly canceled at TE. This is accomplished by using a bilobed read gradient (Figure 7-7).

The first lobe is applied after the 90° pulse but before the measurement process. In fact, it is usually applied prior to the 180° pulse (at the same time as the second lobe of the section select gradient for the 90° pulse). The second lobe of the read gradient is the gradient that is actually on during signal measurement. In order that all phase changes are canceled at TE, the first lobe is of equal magnitude, same direction, and half the duration of the second lobe.

When represented in graphical form, gradients are usually represented by rectangles. The height of the rectangle is proportional to gradient strength and the length is proportional to gradient duration. When the gradient is off, it is represented by a line at the level of the base of the rectangle. A full diagram of a typical spin echo pulse sequence is shown in Figure 7-8.

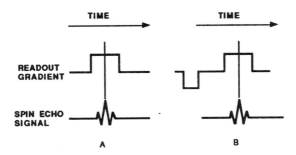

FIGURE 7-7. (A) Readout of the spin echo signal occurs while the readout gradient is on. When the readout gradient is turned on, a phase difference across the section develops. (B) The phase difference can be canceled by the application of a prior gradient, which intentionally dephases the section before the readout gradient. The prior lobe is sometimes referred to as the dephasing lobe.

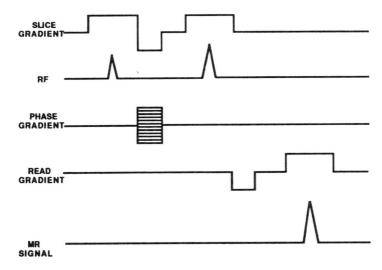

FIGURE 7-8. A schematic diagram of a spin echo pulse sequence. The rectangle with lines along the phase-encoding gradient line is meant to indicate that the phase-encoding gradient is of variable strength.

8 Fourier Analysis, Frequency, Phase, and Signal Sampling

An MR signal is generated by applying an RF pulse to a collection of protons. The total MR signal is equal to the sum of all of the signals emitted by all portions of the collection. In order to generate a useful image, the signal is altered by the application of many gradients. These gradients encode the signal with spatial information. Fourier analysis is then used to decode the signal and determine the individual components. Fourier analysis is based upon the use of periodic functions.

What is a periodic function? A periodic function may be a signal that varies in time, like the voltage in the wires of a circuit that is energized by an alternating current. In the 60-cycle, 110-V alternating current used in the U.S., the voltage varies as shown in Figure 8-1. Here, the voltage is the function f(t) that repeats itself with a time period (T) of 1/60 second. This means that the voltage [f(t)] will have exactly the same value every T interval. In equation form, this is written as

$$f(t) = f(t + T) = f(t + 2T) = f(t + 3T) = \cdots = f(t + nT)$$

for all positive integers n. The equation is very general and can be applied to any periodic function f(t). Over each interval of time of length T, f(t) will go through one complete cycle of values and then repeat. Thus, if f(t) goes through one complete cycle in T seconds, it will go through 1/T cycles in one second. For the alternating current in the U.S., 1/T = 1/(1/60), or 60 cycles per second. The number of cycles per second is customarily called the frequency and is often denoted by ω. Because this is a frequency in time (i.e., the number of cycles **per second**), it is also called a **temporal frequency**. By definition, then, ω = 1/T (i.e., the frequency of a periodic function is equal to the reciprocal of the period and vice versa).

The simplest periodic function is a sinusoidal function such as the sine (sin) or cosine (cos) functions. For example, sin(ωt) is a periodic function of time when t is measured in seconds and ω is measured in radians per second. (A radian is an angular measure equal to 57.296°. By definition, there are 2π radians along the circumference of a circle so that 2π radians equals 360°.) The sine and cosine functions both have a period of 2π radians. (π is the familiar ratio of the circumference of a circle to its diameter, equal to 3.14159 ⋯ .) Thus sin(ωt) = sin(ωt + 2π) = sin(ωt + 4π) = ⋯ sin(ωt + 2nπ) for all integers n. If ω = 1, then the function sin(t) has period 2π seconds and has a frequency equal to 1/2π cycles per second.

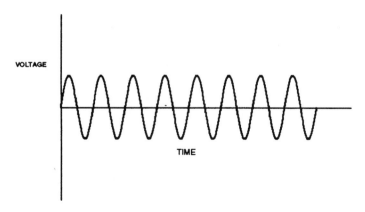

VOLTAGE

TIME

FIGURE 8-1. Voltage varies as a sinusoidal function of time.

What about the function sin(t + π)? This sine function also has period 2π and is identical to the function sin(t) except that the values of sin(t + π) are shifted by a time interval of length π along the time axis (Figure 8-2). These two functions are said to differ in phase by an amount equal to π. It is customary to denote phase by φ. It is important to note that phase is a relative concept. By convention, the function sin(t) is said to be a sine function with phase zero and the function sin(t + φ) is said to be a sine function with phase φ.

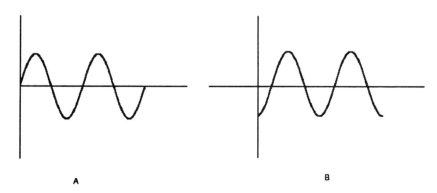

A   B

FIGURE 8-2. The function sin(t) is shown in (A). The function sin(t + π), shown in (B), is identical to sin(t) except that it is shifted along the time axis.

The function cos(t) is said to be a cosine function with phase zero and the function cos(t + φ) is said to be a cosine function with phase φ. In fact, sin(t + π/2) = cos(t). Thus, the cosine function is identical to a sine function, but phase shifted by π/2 (which is equal to 90°). Likewise, cos(t – π/2) = sin(t). Thus, the sine function is identical to a cosine function phase shifted by negative π/2 (i.e., –90°).

Circular motion is an example of a periodic function of time. Suppose a single vector whose base is located at the origin of a Cartesian coordinate system rotates counterclockwise (at a constant velocity) in a circular path (Figure 8-3). If the vector

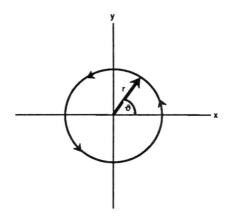

FIGURE 8-3. A vector of length r, rotating counterclockwise in an xy coordinate system.

has length r and at time t it makes an angle ϑ with the positive x axis, then the position of the tip of the vector at time t is given by $x = r\cos\vartheta$ and $y = r\sin\vartheta$. Because the vector rotates at constant velocity, $\vartheta = 2\pi\omega t$, where ω is the angular frequency. Both the x and y coordinates of the vector vary in a sinusoidal manner over time with frequency ω.

Suppose many rotating vectors are located along the x axis, with the base of the n-th vector located at $x = n$ cm, where n is a positive integer (Figure 8-4). Also, suppose the frequency of rotation of each vector depends on the x coordinate such that the frequency of the vector at position n is ωn. The frequency of the vectors, therefore, varies as a function of position (i.e., **spatial** coordinate) along the x axis. The phase of the vectors is assumed to be equal at the time they start rotating. At any given point in time, the frequency is incremented in units of ω cycles per centimeter. This is usually referred to as a **spatial frequency** because it is dependent upon a spatial coordinate. This is identical to a temporal frequency except that the units are cycles per centimeter rather than cycles per second.

In a similar manner, suppose many rotating vectors with angular frequency ω are located along the y axis, with the base of the n-th vector located at $y = n$ cm, where n is a positive integer (Figure 8-5). Also, suppose the phase of each vector is a function of the y coordinate such that the phase of the vector at position n is ϕn. The phase of the vectors then varies as a function of position along the y axis and is incremented in units of ϕ cycles per centimeter. This is also a spatial frequency. The units are identical to the spatial frequency described in the paragraph above. Therefore, we see that a spatial variation of frequency (with constant phase) is exactly equivalent to a spatial variation of phase (with constant frequency).

Just as ω is used to denote temporal frequencies, k is customarily used to denote spatial frequencies. Furthermore, if the spatial coordinate is the x coordinate, the symbol k_x is usually used to denote the spatial frequency. Likewise, if the spatial coordinate is the y coordinate, the symbol k_y is usually used to denote the spatial frequency. The coordinate system formed by the k_x and k_y axes is usually referred to as k space (Figure 8-6).

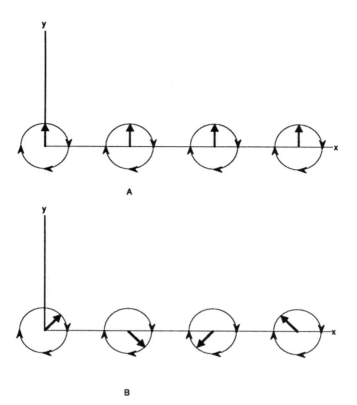

FIGURE 8-4 A & B. The rotating vectors have a different frequency, dependent on their position on the x axis. When viewed at a given point in time, the frequency differences cause the vectors to be out of phase. When viewed over time, the phase differences change. At top (A), all of the vectors are in phase. A short time later (B), a phase difference has developed.

When a collection of protons is excited by an RF pulse, longitudinal magnetization within each voxel is converted into transverse magnetization. The transverse magnetization within each voxel then rotates around the axis of the external magnetic field (like a rotating vector). These rotating magnetic vectors induce a signal (i.e., an electric voltage) in the receiver coil. This signal varies as a function of time. Unfortunately, this signal represents the sum of all of the signals from all of the voxels. The purpose of the MRI process is to determine the signal originating from the individual voxels. The magnitude of the signal from each voxel is proportional to the net transverse magnetization within the voxel.

The MR signal is spatially encoded by the application of the frequency- and phase-encoding gradients. These gradients encode the signal by introducing spatial variations of frequency and phase along two perpendicular directions. This is identical to the rotating vectors in Figures 8-4 and 8-5, which vary in frequency along the x axis and vary in phase along the y axis. Spatial "decoding" of the MR signal is accomplished by using Fourier analysis, which will be described next.

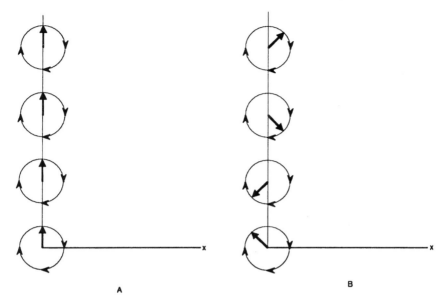

FIGURE 8-5 A & B. All vectors initially have the same frequency and phase (A). In (B), the phase has been altered as a function of position along the y axis. These phase changes will persist over time. Note the similarity between 8-4 B and 8-5 B. A frequency difference viewed at a single point in time is equivalent to a phase difference.

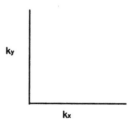

FIGURE 8-6. The coordinate system formed by the k_x and k_y axes, referred to as "k space."

The analysis of the temporal changes in a signal is an important application of Fourier analysis. This mathematical tool is widely used in medical imaging, and is fundamental to understanding MRI. Fourier analysis involves combining many sine functions in an attempt to reproduce an observed or experimental function. Fourier analysis also works in reverse: given a time-varying signal, it is possible to determine what frequencies are present in the signal. For example, if hourly temperature readings were recorded over a period of one year at one location in the northern hemisphere, Fourier analysis would be able to pick out both the daily and the annual temperature variations, which have periods of one day and one year, respectively.

We now look at a more difficult problem. Consider the square wave function of time shown in Figure 8-7. This function is defined by the equation f(t) = −1 when −1/2 < t < 0, f(t) = 1 when 0 < t < 1/2, and f(t) = f(t + 1). The function sin2πt serves as a reasonable first approximation to f(t). It is a good approximation near the center of each square wave but is a poor approximation near the edges. What if we add the functions sin2πt and (1/3)sin(6πt)? The function sin2πt + (1/3)sin6πt gives a better approximation of the square wave function than does sin2πt, especially at the edges.

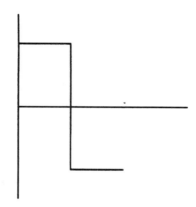

FIGURE 8-7.   One cycle of the square wave function.

Suppose we add the functions sin2πt, (1/3)sin6πt, and (1/5)sin10πt? This gives an even better approximation to the square wave function, especially at the edges. Note that the amplitudes (1/3) and (1/5) of the higher frequency functions are smaller than the fundamental sin2πt function. In fact, if we continue to add sine functions of higher frequency and lower amplitude, we will obtain a better and better approximation to the square wave function (Figures 8-8 and 8-9).

Thus, we see that the higher amplitude (and lower frequency) sine waves primarily provide the overall amplitude of the approximation, especially near the center of the square wave. The lower amplitude (and higher frequency) sine waves primarily provide the fine detail needed at the edges of the approximation. In fact, it can be shown mathematically that the square wave function under discussion can be exactly duplicated as the sum of the following series of sine terms: sin(2πt) + (1/3)sin(6πt) + (1/5)sin(10πt) + ⋯ + (1/n)sin(2nπt) + ⋯ + , for all positive odd integers n. As higher frequency, lower amplitude sine functions are added to the series, they change the overall amplitude very little but continue to smooth the edges of the approximation.

In fact, it can be shown mathematically that any well-behaved periodic function can be expressed as a sum of sine and cosine functions. Suppose f(t) is any periodic function of time of period T and frequency ω. The n-th term of such a sum will contain sine and cosine functions of the form sin(2πnωt) and cos(2πnωt). These sine and cosine functions have frequency nω.

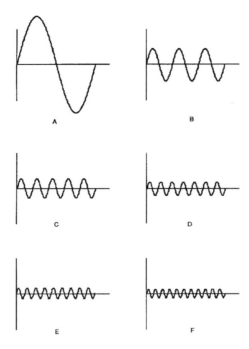

FIGURE 8-8. (**A**) sin(t). (**B**) (1/3)sin(3t). (**C**) (1/5)sin(5t) (**D**) (1/7)sin(7t). (**E**) (1/9)sin(9t). (**F**) (1/11)sin(11t).

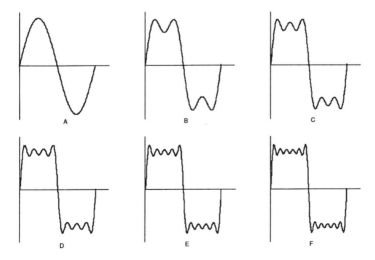

FIGURE 8-9. (**A**) sin(t). (**B**) sin(t) + (1/3)sin(3t). (**C**) sin(t) + (1/3)sin(3t) + (1/5)sin(5t). (**D**) sin(t) + (1/3)sin(3t) + (1/5)sin(5t) + (1/7)sin(7t). (**E**) sin(t) + (1/3)sin(3t) + (1/5)sin(5t) + (1/7)sin(7t) + (1/9)sin(9t). (**F**) sin(t) + (1/3)sin(3t) + (1/5)sin(5t) + (1/7)sin(7t) + (1/9)sin(9t) + (1/11)sin(11t).

This means that any periodic function of frequency ω can be represented by a sum of sine and cosine functions of frequencies equal to integral multiples of the frequency of the periodic function itself. The amplitude of each sine and cosine function in the sum will vary depending upon f(t). In general, the amplitude of each sine and cosine function will decrease as its frequency increases. It is customary to denote the amplitudes of the sine and cosine functions $\sin(2\pi n\omega t)$ and $\cos(2\pi n\omega t)$ as A_n and B_n, respectively. The subscript n for these coefficients indicates that they are a function of the frequency $n\omega$.

Mathematically, a sum of terms is usually referred to simply as a series. When a periodic function is expressed as a sum of sine and cosine functions, it is referred to as a **Fourier series**. The amplitudes of the sine and cosine functions (A_n and B_n) are referred to as the **Fourier coefficients**. Without going into the mathematical details, if a function is known, the Fourier coefficients can be computed using a standard formula. Likewise, if the Fourier series of a function is known, the function itself can be determined (usually referred to as taking the inverse Fourier transform).

What about nonperiodic functions? Suppose a function g(t) is nonzero over a finite interval of time (say, from t = 0 to t = T) and is zero for all values of t outside this interval. We can form the periodic function f(t) that is equal to g(t) over every interval of length T. We can then compute the Fourier series of f(t) and this will equal g(t) over the interval from t = 0 to t = T. In fact, even if g(t) is not zero outside of the interval t = 0 to t = T, the Fourier series of f(t) can be used to compute g(t) over this interval. In this way, we can even compute the Fourier series of a nonperiodic function over any finite interval.

Suppose we let the interval t = 0 to t = T get very large. That is, suppose T is very large. This corresponds to $\omega = 1/T$ being very small. This means that the difference in frequency between consecutive terms of the Fourier series will be very small because this difference equals ω. Such a sum becomes an integral. Thus, if we let the period of a function become infinite (i.e., the function is not periodic), the Fourier series becomes an integral. This integral is referred to as the **Fourier integral**.

What does it mean when the period of a function is infinite (which is equivalent to a frequency of zero)? Since the period of a function is the interval after which the function repeats itself, a function with infinite period no longer repeats itself. That is, a function with infinite period is no longer periodic. Every nonperiodic function is essentially a function of infinite period. Thus, although we cannot represent a nonperiodic function by a Fourier series, we can represent any nonperiodic function by a Fourier integral. In fact, the Fourier integral of a periodic function reduces to a Fourier series.

A Fourier series expresses a periodic function as a discrete sum of sine and cosine functions. By discrete is meant that the frequencies of the sine and cosine functions in the sum are incremented by a finite amount between consecutive terms of the sum. The Fourier coefficients give the amplitudes of each of the sine and cosine functions at each frequency. If the periodic function is of frequency ω, then the sine and cosine functions in the sum have frequencies $n\omega$ for all positive integers n.

The Fourier integral of a function expresses the function as a continuous sum (in the form of an integral) of sine and cosine functions. Analogous to the Fourier coefficients, the amplitude of each of the sine and cosine functions is referred to as the Fourier transform. The **Fourier transform** is a continuous function of frequency.

Suppose we wish to determine the Fourier transform of a nonperiodic function of time f(t). Use the symbol F to denote the Fourier transform. The Fourier transform of a function of time gives the amplitude of the sine and cosine functions as a function of **temporal** frequency, namely $F(\omega)$. Thus, the Fourier transform of a function of time is a function of temporal frequency. Examples are shown in Figure 8-10. Likewise, the Fourier transform of a nonperiodic function of position gives the amplitude of the sine and cosine functions as a function of **spatial** frequency. Since it is customary to use k to denote spatial frequency, the Fourier transform of a function of position is usually written as F(k).

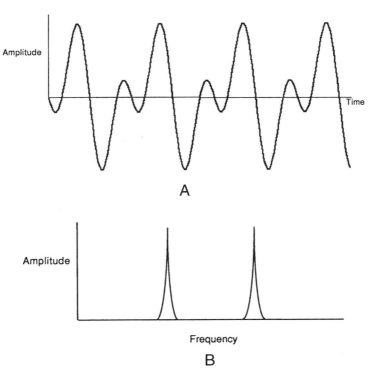

FIGURE 8-10 A & B. Examples of the Fourier transform. (A) and (B) show the function sin(t) + sin(2t) and its Fourier transform, respectively. The Fourier transform shows two discrete values corresponding to the two frequencies of sin(t) and sin(2t). In this sense, the Fourier transform of a periodic function of time simply yields the amplitudes of the different frequency components (i.e., amplitude as a function of frequency). The function sin(t) + sin(2t) has two frequency components of equal amplitude, shown by the two spikes in (B).

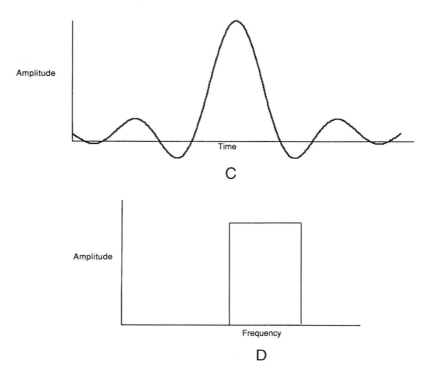

FIGURE 8-10 C & D. (C) and (D) show the function sin(t)/t and its Fourier transform, respectively.

To summarize, then, any (well-behaved) function can be expressed as a Fourier integral. An integral is simply an infinite sum. In the case of the Fourier integral, it is a sum of sine and cosine functions of different frequency. The amplitude of the sine and cosine functions in the sum is given by the Fourier transform. If the function happens to be periodic, then the Fourier integral reduces to a Fourier series and the Fourier transform reduces to the Fourier coefficients. The Fourier series is therefore a special case of the Fourier transform. In the remainder of the discussion we will therefore use the term Fourier transform (which includes Fourier series as a special case).

How does one actually compute the Fourier transform of a function? If the precise mathematical form of the function is known, there are standard formulas that can be used to directly calculate the Fourier transform. However, in many practical applications we will need to compute the Fourier transform of a measured function whose precise mathematical form is unknown. For example, the MR signal is detected as a voltage induced in a receiver coil. Although the voltage is readily measured as a function of time, its precise mathematical formula is unknown.

The MR signal is an analog signal. By definition, an analog signal is a continuous function of time. In order for a computer to be able to analyze this signal, it must convert the analog signal into a digital signal. A digital signal is a discrete function of time. By definition, a discrete function of time assumes only a finite number of values at specific points of time (Figure 8-11).

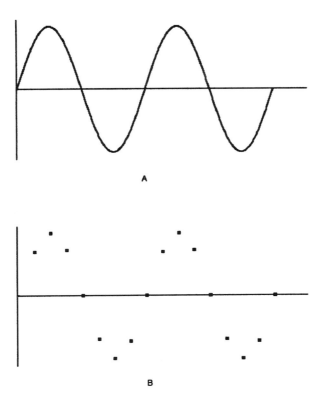

A

B

FIGURE 8-11. (A) An analog signal is represented by a continuous sine wave. (B) Discrete values of the sine wave are the digital representation of the function shown in (A).

Why can't a computer directly analyze a continuous signal? In order to analyze a signal, a computer must store the measured values of the signal; that is, a number. A continuous signal has an infinite number of values, even over the shortest interval of time. It is impossible for a computer to store an infinite number of values. Instead, the computer measures the signal at a finite number of closely spaced specific points in time and uses these values as a representation of the signal. Each such signal measurement takes a small amount of time to perform. The maximum rate at which signal measurements can be made is limited by the time it takes to perform each measurement.

The conversion of an analog signal into a digital signal is performed by an analog-to-digital converter (ADC). Suppose we wish to digitize the continuous function of time $V(t)$, where V stands for voltage. We measure $V(t)$ at n equally spaced discrete points of time denoted by t_1, t_2, t_3, $\cdots$, t_n. This yields the series of signal measurements $V(t_1)$, $V(t_2)$, $V(t_3)$, $\cdots$, $V(t_n)$. This is the computer representation of the signal V(t). Each signal measurement is referred to as a sample. The time between samples is referred to as the sampling interval (denoted by Δt). The total time over which samples are taken is referred to as the sampling time (T_s). Note that $T_s = n\Delta t$.

How can we ensure the accuracy of the digital representation of an analog signal? The MR signal consists of many sinusoidal components that have different frequencies and phases. Let's look at the accuracy of the digital representation of a single sinusoidal function such as $\sin(2\pi\omega t)$. This function has frequency ω. By definition, this function is periodic and goes through ω cycles every second. Hence, the time of one cycle (i.e., the period) is $1/\omega$ seconds.

The function $\sin(-2\pi\omega t)$ also has frequency ω but advances through its cycles in an opposite manner with respect to the function $\sin(2\pi\omega t)$. By convention, the function $\sin(2\pi\omega t)$ advances through its cycles in a positive manner and the function $\sin(-2\pi\omega t)$ advances through its cycles in a negative manner. In fact, $\sin(-2\pi\omega t) = \sin(2\pi\omega t + \pi)$, which means that these two functions are identical except that they are 180° (or π radians) out of phase.

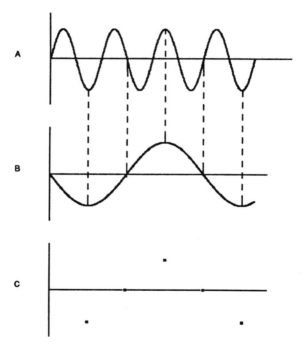

FIGURE 8-12. (A) Samples of the function $\sin(2\pi\omega t)$ are taken at the points indicated along the dashed lines. (B) Samples of the function $\sin(-2\pi\omega t/3)$ at the same points in time as those shown in (A) are identical. (C) The digital representation of both functions is the same.

How often must a signal be sampled to ensure that the ADC process provides an accurate representation of the actual signal? It turns out that if a function advances through more than one-half cycle between samplings, then its frequency cannot be accurately determined by the ADC process. Another way to say this is that the signal must be sampled at least twice per cycle in order to get the right answer from the Fourier analysis.

For example, suppose we sample the function $\sin(2\pi\omega t)$ at intervals of 3/4 of a cycle. This would require sampling every $3/4\omega$ seconds. The function $\sin(-2\pi\omega t/3)$ advances through its cycles one-third as fast as the function $\sin(2\pi\omega t)$ but in the opposite direction. In $3/4\omega$ seconds, the function $\sin(-2\pi\omega t/3)$ will advance through 1/4 of a negative cycle. But 3/4 positive cycles is equal to 1/4 negative cycles. Therefore, the functions $\sin(2\pi\omega t)$ and $\sin(-2\pi\omega t/3)$ will have identical values every $3/4\omega$ seconds. Therefore, if samples are taken every $3/4\omega$ seconds, one cannot distinguish between the function $\sin(2\omega t)$ and the function $\sin(-2\pi\omega t/3)$ (Figure 8-12).

The above result is usually referred to as the **Nyquist theorem**. This theorem states that if a signal consisting of many frequency components is digitized, it must be sampled at a rate equal to at least twice the highest frequency component in the signal.

The Fourier transform of the function V(t) described above can be closely approximated, based upon the sample values used to digitize the voltage. Because it is based upon the discrete sample values, it is usually referred to as a **discrete Fourier transform**.

What does all this have to do with MRI? Following the section selective excitation pulse, transverse magnetization is created within a section of tissue. The section can be thought of as consisting of many small volume elements (voxels). At the time of signal measurement, each voxel will contain a unique amount of transverse magnetization. The amount of transverse magnetization (within each voxel) is dependent upon the T1, T2, and proton density of the tissue contained within the voxel. Denote the transverse magnetization at the time of signal measurement within the voxel centered at the point (x,y) as M(x,y). The signal arising from this voxel is directly proportional to M(x,y).

The sole purpose of the imaging process is to determine the function M(x,y) and to represent it in the MR image as a picture element (pixel), the brightness of which is proportional to M(x,y). Unfortunately, M(x,y) cannot be measured directly. The MRI process converts M(x,y) into a corresponding voltage in the receiver coil. The Fourier transform of the voltage is then used to compute the function M(x,y) itself. How is this achieved?

Following an excitation pulse, transverse magnetization within each voxel rotates around the B_0 field. Due to its precessional motion, the transverse magnetization within each voxel induces a voltage in the receiver coil that is directly proportional to M(x,y). The rotational motion can therefore be thought of as converting M(x,y) into a voltage in the receiver coil. The total (or net) voltage induced by all voxels can be directly measured as a function of time. Denote the net voltage at time t as V(t).

The effect of the precessional motion of the transverse magnetization therefore converts the function M(x,y) into a function of time, V(t). The signal measurement process is repeated many times, each time with a different strength phase-encoding gradient (denoted by G_n for the n-th signal measurement). The induced voltage following the n-th excitation is therefore more accurately denoted by $V(t,G_n)$.

In addition to amplitude, the voltage induced in the receiver coil by the transverse magnetization of each voxel also has a phase. Immediately following an excitation pulse, transverse magnetization within all voxels will have the same phase. Since phase is a relative term, the phase of the signal from each voxel must be defined with respect to some reference signal. In fact, the reference signal used by the MRI system is a signal at the resonance frequency. The phase of the reference can be arbitrarily chosen, but once selected, the phase of all signals is defined with respect to the phase of the reference.

In converting $M(x,y)$ into $V(t,G_n)$, we have lost all spatial encoding. Although the $M(x,y)$ of each voxel will induce a voltage in the receiver coil that is proportional to the amount of transverse magnetization within the voxel, we can measure only the total voltage induced by all voxels. Therefore, how can we use $V(t)$ to determine individual $M(x,y)$ values? If we can somehow spatially encode the voltage induced in the receiver coil by each $M(x,y)$ for each individual excitation, then we should be able to determine $M(x,y)$. In fact, it is the frequency- and phase-encoding gradients that spatially encode the measured voltage. How is this achieved?

The frequency of rotation of the transverse magnetization in a given voxel is determined by the local field strength. If the local field strength at all points is B_0 (the strength of the main magnetic field), then all transverse magnetization will rotate at the frequency $\omega_0 = \gamma B_0$, which is precisely the resonance frequency.

Suppose we apply a linear gradient (change the B_0 field) along the x axis during the voltage measurement such that the local field strength at the point (x,y) differs from B_0 by Gx, where G is a constant (namely, the amplitude of the gradient). G is in units of change in magnetic field strength per unit distance along the x axis (i.e., gauss per centimeter). In the presence of this gradient, transverse magnetization at the point (x,y) will precess at a frequency that differs from the resonance frequency by γGx (note that γGx is in units of cycles per second). This gradient is precisely the read (or frequency-encoding) gradient of a standard imaging sequence.

As previously noted, the voltage is an analog signal that varies with time. In order to analyze the signal voltage, we measure (i.e., sample) it at discrete points of time t. The time of each signal sample is usually defined with respect to the center of the frequency-encoding gradient. If T_S is the total sampling time, then signal samples are obtained from time $t = -T_S/2$ to $t = T_S/2$, and $t = 0$ corresponds to the center of the frequency-encoding gradient. The frequency-encoding gradient is bilobed such that all phase changes it induces are canceled at the center of the gradient (see Figure 7-5). It is for this reason that time is defined as $t = 0$ at the center of the frequency-encoding gradient.

With the read gradient on, when a measurement of the induced voltage is obtained at time t, we can think of the transverse magnetization within each voxel as having a frequency that is higher or lower than the reference signal (which is at the resonance frequency). The frequency difference is a function of position along the x axis and is given by γGx. This is a spatial frequency because it is expressed as a number that depends on the location along the x axis. Therefore, the voltage at time t corresponds to a spatial frequency equal to γGx along the x axis. This spatial frequency is usually denoted by the variable k_x (i.e., $k_x = \gamma Gx$), and the corresponding voltage can be denoted by $V(k_x)$.

If nothing else were done and the Fourier transform of $V(t)$ was computed, it would yield the amplitude of the different temporal frequency components of the voltage. Each temporal frequency component in turn corresponds to a different x coordinate. A temporal frequency component that differs from the resonance frequency by an amount $\Delta \omega$ corresponds to the x coordinate $\Delta \omega / \gamma G$. Alternatively, we can compute the Fourier transform of $V(k_x)$. This would yield the amplitude of the signal as a function of the x coordinate directly (since k_x converts a function of time into a function of position). We could therefore determine the total amplitude of transverse magnetization with a given x coordinate.

However, we still need to determine position along the y axis. How is this achieved? Suppose that prior to the read gradient (and therefore prior to the voltage measurement) we turn on (for a short time) a second linear gradient, this time along the y axis. Suppose the strength of this gradient at point (x,y) is Hy (where H is some constant) and that the gradient is on for time t. After this gradient is turned off, transverse magnetization at the point (x,y) will rotate at a phase that differs from the reference signal by γHty. This gradient is equivalent to the phase-encoding gradient of a standard imaging sequence.

The larger the time t and/or the greater the value of H, the greater the phase change induced in a given voxel by the phase-encoding gradient. However, the phase-encoding gradient strength is different following each excitation. This is usually accomplished by keeping the time t unchanged and incrementing the value of H by a constant amount (ΔH) between phase-encoding steps. A common scheme is to move in sequential fashion from the most negative to the most positive gradient. The n-th phase-encoding gradient, G_n, will then have strength $G_n = (k - n - 1)\Delta H$, where $k = 1$ to $2n$.

Following each excitation and phase encoding with each fixed value of G_n, the coil output voltage is sampled at times $t = -T_S/2$ to $t = T_S/2$. In a similar manner, phase samples are obtained at different phase-encoding gradient strengths (G_n) for each fixed value of t. At the time of each phase sample, the transverse magnetization within each voxel can be thought of as having gone through a certain number of additional or fewer cycles with respect to the phase of the reference signal. The number of additional or fewer cycles is now a function of position along the y axis as well as the phase-encoding gradient increment (ΔH). The number of cycles per centimeter (following G_n) is given by $\gamma n\Delta Ht$ (remember, ΔH is in units of gauss per centimeter, so that $\gamma n\Delta H$ is in units of [cycles per second] per centimeter and $\gamma n\Delta Ht$ is in units of cycles per centimeter). This is a **spatial frequency**.

Therefore, the voltage at time t following phase-encoding gradient G_n corresponds to the spatial frequency $\gamma n\Delta Ht$ along the y axis. This spatial frequency is usually denoted by the variable k_y (i.e., $k_y = \gamma n\Delta Ht$), and the corresponding voltage can be denoted as $V(k_y)$.

The signal originating at each y coordinate undergoes a unique (incremental) phase change with respect to the reference from one phase-encoding gradient to the next (namely, $\gamma \Delta Hty$). Therefore, any signal undergoing an incremental phase change of $\Delta\phi$ between phase-encoding gradients corresponds to the y coordinate $\Delta\phi/\gamma\Delta Ht$.

The effect of using both the frequency- and phase-encoding gradients, then, is to cause the net induced voltage to consist of a superposition of voltages at different frequency and phase. Each voltage measurement corresponds to a different spatial frequency along the k_x and k_y axes and the voltage can be denoted by $V(k_x,k_y)$. If we take the Fourier transform of $V(k_x,k_y)$, we can determine $M(x,y)$.

The coordinate system with axes k_x and k_y is usually referred to as **k space**. The greater the value of k_x, the greater the corresponding spatial frequency along the k_x axis. The greater the value of k_y, the greater the corresponding spatial frequency along the k_y axis. The higher spatial frequencies correspond to the higher frequency sine and cosine functions in the Fourier transform of $M(x,y)$. The lower spatial frequencies correspond to the lower frequency sine and cosine functions in the Fourier transform of $M(x,y)$.

Therefore, the stronger phase-encoding gradients correspond to the Fourier coefficients of $M(x,y)$ of the higher spatial frequency components along the y axis. Likewise, the weaker phase-encoding gradients correspond to the Fourier coefficients of $M(x,y)$ of the lower spatial frequency components along the y axis Therefore, the signal from measurements obtained with the stronger phase-encoding gradients provides mainly fine detail information (i.e., spatial resolution) and the signal from measurements obtained with the weaker phase-encoding gradients provides mainly signal intensity and thus contrast information. These points are important in understanding fast spin echo imaging and will be discussed in Chapter 11.

9 Signal-to-Noise Ratio

Consider any measurement process that has an outcome expressed as a number (or value). Denote the outcome of a single measurement as M. If the measurement is repeated many times the value of M will not always be the same. It will vary somewhat around a mean (or average) value. The mean value of M is usually denoted by μ. The variability around the average value is expressed by the standard deviation. The standard deviation is defined mathematically as the square root of the mean value of $(M - \mu)^2$ and the standard deviation is usually denoted by σ. The greater the value of the standard deviation, the more variability there is in each individual measurement.

Suppose we repeat a measurement process n times and denote the outcome of the n-th measurement as M_n. If we define A_n as $A_n = (M_1 + M_2 + \cdots + M_n)/n$, then A_n is the average of the n measurements. If each individual measurement has mean value μ and standard deviation σ, it can be shown mathematically that the mean of A_n is μ and the standard deviation of A_n is $\sigma\sqrt{n}$. The effect of using the average value of multiple measurements is to reduce the standard deviation by a factor proportional to the square root of the number of measurements, while leaving the mean unchanged. Therefore, if we use the average value of many measurements, we reduce the variability of the outcome. This makes intuitive sense. Each individual measurement will be greater than, less than, or equal to the mean. By adding many measurements, the values greater than or less than the mean will cancel out to some degree (depending on the number of measurements).

When performing MRI, one measures a signal many times. This signal will have some variability due to the superimposition of noise. Noise arises from many sources, including random electric currents in the patient as well as random electric currents within resistive elements of the receiver. This type of noise is of approximately equal intensity over a wide range of frequencies, and so is referred to as white noise (just as white light consists of light of all frequencies). Because noise is completely random, it will cause both increases and decreases in the observed signal intensity for each individual measurement. The standard deviation of the signal intensity is a measure of the noise. In fact, the standard deviation of the signal intensity of the air surrounding an object being imaged is equal to the noise in the image.

It is now easy to understand the effect of performing many signal measurements on the signal-to-noise ratio (S/N) of an MR image. Suppose n signal measurements are performed and that M_n is the amplitude of the n-th signal measurement. The S/N is then equal to $A_n / (\sigma\sqrt{n})$, which equals $(\sqrt{n})A_n / \sigma$. Therefore, the S/N of an MR image is proportional to the square root of the total number of signal measurements.

When obtaining an MR image, what is the total number of signal measurements? At least one signal measurement must be performed for each phase-encoding gradient. The number of phase-encoding gradients is equal to the size of the phase matrix (denoted as N_p). For each phase-encoding gradient, many excitations can be performed. By definition, the number of excitations per phase-encoding gradient is referred to as the number of signal averages (denoted by NSA). Therefore, the total number of signal measurements is equal to $N_p \times$ NSA, and the S/N is proportional to $\sqrt{(Np \times NSA)}$.

Other factors also affect the S/N of an MR image. The signal that makes up an MR image arises from the protons excited by the RF pulse. The total signal arises from all of the individual voxels in the imaging volume. The imaging process determines the signal intensity arising from each individual voxel. These signal intensities are then assigned to the appropriate picture elements (or pixels) in the final image display.

The sum of all signals from all voxels equals the total signal. For a given imaging sequence and for a given section of tissue, this total is a constant. If all other factors are equal (i.e., tissue T1, T2, and proton density, etc.) the amount of signal arising from a given voxel is proportional to voxel size (or volume). How can voxel volume be calculated?

The field of view (FOV) represents the physical length along both encoding directions from which signal is derived for a given image. Only anatomy contained within the physical boundaries of the FOV will contribute signal to the final image (assuming no wraparound). The FOV is commonly denoted by a single number because it is usually a square, although a rectangular FOV can also be used.

Let L_f be the length of the FOV along the frequency-encoding direction and let L_p be the length of the FOV along the phase-encoding direction. If the number of frequency encodings is N_f and the number of phase encodings is N_p, then the length of each voxel along the frequency-encoding direction is L_f/N_f, and the length of each voxel along the phase encoding direction is L_p/N_p. If the thickness of the section of tissue being imaged is T, then the volume of each voxel is equal to $(L_f/N_f) \times (L_p/N_p) \times T$. This is equal to $[L_f \times L_p \times T]/(N_p \times N_f)$.

Therefore, taking both voxel volume and the number of signal measurements into account, S/N is proportional to $[\sqrt{(N_p \times NSA)}] \times [L_f x L_p \times T]/(N_p \times N_f)]$. Simplification of this expression yields $[L_f \times L_p \times T] \times (\sqrt{NSA})/[N_f \times (\sqrt{N_p})]$. That is, the S/N is directly proportional to the lengths of the FOV, directly proportional to the section thickness, directly proportional to the square root of the NSA, inversely proportional to the number of frequency encodings, and inversely proportional to the square root of the number of phase encodings.

The above expression shows that there is less penalty in S/N for doubling the phase matrix size than doubling the frequency matrix size. Although doubling the phase matrix size will decrease voxel volume by one half, it will also double the total number of excitations. On the other hand, doubling of the frequency matrix size only has the effect of reducing voxel volume by one half.

One additional factor must be considered. So far we have assumed that all of the noise within the imaging volume is superimposed on the MR signal. However, virtually all scanners routinely employ a frequency filter. This filter allows only a narrow band of frequencies to reach the receiver. The band of frequencies is exactly equal to those present within the signal. If the frequency-encoding gradient induces a bandwidth of ±16 kHz across the FOV, then only frequencies within the range

(63.87 MHz ± 16 kHz) will reach the receiver. Therefore, only noise within this same frequency range can reach the receiver.

If we assume that the noise is evenly distributed among all frequencies, then changing the signal bandwidth will affect the noise content of the image. It can be shown mathematically that S/N is inversely proportional to the square root of the sampling time. That is, S/N is proportional to $1 / \sqrt{[\text{Sampling Time}]}$. The square root that occurs in this formula arises from the same formula used above for the standard deviation of multiple measurements. How does this come about?

When the MR signal is measured, in order to avoid aliasing, samples are taken at a rate equal to at least twice the highest frequency component in the signal. In this context, frequency components are defined with respect to the resonance (or reference) frequency. If the MR signal contains frequencies within the range (63.87 MHz ± 16 kHz), then the sampling rate is 32 kHz, which means that 32,000 samples are taken per second. The time between samples is therefore equal to 1/32,000 s, which equals 1/32 ms.

On most imaging systems, the sampling rate would be chosen to equal 32 kHz (rather than a greater sampling rate). The sampling time (T_S) is equal to the total number of samples multiplied by the time between samples. The total number of samples is equal to the size of the frequency matrix (N_f). If $N_f = 256$, and the sampling rate is 32 kHz, then T_S will equal 1/32 ms multiplied by 256, which equals 8 ms.

Consider an MRI sequence performed with a signal bandwidth of ±16 kHz, $N_f = 256$, and the sampling rate equal to 32 kHz. The highest frequency component in the signal will go through one-half cycle (with respect to the resonance frequency) between samples. Lower frequency components will go through less than one-half cycle between samples (with the lowest frequency component not advancing at all). The average number of cycles through which all of the frequency components advance between samples is one-quarter cycle (halfway between 0 and 1/2).

What about the noise? Noise is a random process superimposed on the signal. If the noise is in phase with the signal it will cause it to increase. If the noise is out of phase with the signal it will cause it to decrease. This does not affect the mean value of the signal intensity (because half of the time the noise increases the signal and half of the time it decreases the signal), but it does affect the standard deviation of the signal intensity. The effect of doing multiple signal measurements is to improve the S/N by "averaging out" the noise.

In an identical manner, the more cycles each frequency component of a signal goes through during the measurement process, the more the noise will be averaged out. If all other factors are held constant, the S/N is proportional to the square root of the average number of cycles through which the frequency components of the signal advance during the measurement process. For a given signal bandwidth, the number of cycles advanced between samples will be maximized by using the minimum sampling rate (i.e., sampling at twice the highest frequency component). For a fixed size of the frequency matrix, T_S is inversely proportional to the sampling rate. Therefore, for a given signal bandwidth and frequency matrix size, the S/N is inversely proportional to the square root of T_S.

Taking all of the factors discussed thus far into account, S/N is proportional to $[L_f \times L_p] \times T \times (\sqrt{NSA}) \times (\sqrt{T_S})/[(N_f \times (\sqrt{N_p})]$.

The sampling time (T_S) is determined by the sampling rate and the total number of frequency samples (N_f). For the reasons previously discussed, on most imaging systems, the sampling rate is equal to twice the signal bandwidth (BW). Therefore, $T_S = N_f/BW$. For a fixed value of N_f, T_S will be maximized by minimizing BW.

As previously noted, the standard (or default) signal bandwidth on most imaging systems is ±16 kHz. Why not use a narrower signal bandwidth in order to increase T_s and improve S/N? The reason is that there are significant penalties for using a narrow signal bandwidth. These will be discussed separately.

The total sampling time is equal to the product of the total number of frequency samples and the time per sample. The time per sample is the reciprocal of the sampling rate. The sampling rate is equal to twice the signal bandwidth. Assuming $N_f = 256$, for a ±32-kHz signal bandwidth, the sampling time is $[256 \times (1/64000)]$ $T_S = 4$ ms. For a ±16-kHz signal bandwidth, the sampling time is 8 ms. For a ±8-kHz signal bandwidth, the sampling time is 16 ms. For a ±4=kHz signal bandwidth, the sampling time is $[256 \times (1/8,000)]$, or 32 ms. In general, if the signal bandwidth is ±b kHz, the sampling time is 128/b ms.

When an MR signal is measured, the read gradient must be on during the entire sampling process. A spin echo is measured such that the center of the read gradient occurs at the echo time (TE). The earliest that the read gradient can possibly be turned on is immediately after the 180° refocusing pulse has been applied. Let the 180° refocusing pulse of a spin echo sequence be applied at time t_1 after a 90° pulse and let the read gradient be turned on at the same time as the 180° pulse. If the read gradient has duration T_S milliseconds, then the center of the read gradient will occur after the read gradient has been on for $T_S/2$ milliseconds. By definition, a spin echo will occur at time $2t_1$. But $2t_1$ must equal $t_1 + T_S/2$, which means that $t_1 = T_S/2$. Therefore, the earliest possible time that a spin echo can occur is $2t_1 = T_S$ milliseconds.

For example, when using a ±16-kHz bandwidth, the sampling time is 8 ms and the minimum TE would be 8 ms. When using a ±4-kHz bandwidth, the sampling time is 32 ms and the minimum TE is also 32 ms. In addition, when using a ±4-kHz bandwidth, the longer readout period will decrease the number of sections that can be acquired, because more time will be spent measuring the signal in each section. Therefore, the penalty for using a narrower bandwidth is an increase in the minimum TE and a reduction in the number of sections that can be acquired.

A second problem that arises when using a narrow bandwidth is worsening of chemical shift artifact. At 1.5 T, lipid protons precess at a frequency 220 Hz lower than water protons. Position along the frequency-encoding direction is determined by frequency. The imaging system has to assume that all protons within a sample are in water (or that all are in lipid). Usually, the former assumption is made, because the majority of tissue protons are in water. Therefore, since the scanner assumes that all protons are in water, the position of lipid protons along the frequency-encoding direction will be misregistered (this will be discussed in greater detail in Chapters 10 and 14).

The degree of misregistration is dependent on the signal bandwidth. When the bandwidth across the field of view is ±16 kHz, the total frequency change across the field of view along the frequency direction is 32 kHz. If the size of the frequency matrix is 256, then the frequency change per pixel is equal to (32,000/256) Hz, which equals 125 Hz per pixel. Therefore, the position of lipid protons will be misregistered by (220/125) = 1.75 pixels. The position will be shifted toward the direction of decreasing frequency.

If the bandwidth is ±4 kHz, the frequency change per pixel along the frequency-encoding direction is 8000/256, which equals 31.25 Hz per pixel. In this case the position of lipid protons is misregistered by (220/31.25) = 7 pixels. Therefore, another penalty for using a narrower bandwidth is worsening of chemical shift artifact along the frequency-encoding direction.

It is, therefore, apparent that although use of a narrower bandwidth will result in improved S/N, there are significant penalties associated with it that must be considered. The standard (default) bandwidth of ±16 kHz is chosen as a compromise.

10 Imaging Options

Performing an MRI examination requires that the user choose from among a large number of imaging parameters and optional imaging features. Optional imaging features often serve to eliminate image artifacts and image degradation that can arise from motion, blood flow, cardiac activity, etc. The ability to choose the appropriate imaging parameters and options requires an understanding of how they work.

1 REDUCTION OF MOTION-INDUCED GHOST ARTIFACTS

Regardless of the imaging sequence, inadvertent patient movement as well as physiologic motion will lead to artifacts. Physiologic motion includes respiratory motion, vascular pulsation, blood flow, and cardiac motion. The most troublesome artifact associated with motion of any type is ghost artifact.

1.1 ORIGIN OF GHOST ARTIFACT

As noted in Chapter 8, the sole purpose of the MRI process is to determine the value of $M(x,y)$ (the transverse magnetization) within all of the voxels of a section of tissue. This is accomplished by performing many successive selective excitations of the section, each with a different strength phase-encoding gradient. After excitation and phase-encoding, the signal (a time-varying voltage induced in the receiver coil) is read out while the frequency-encoding gradient is on. The Fourier transform of the induced voltage signals (recorded as digital values in k space) yields the values of $M(x,y)$. These computations assume that the tissue content of each voxel remains constant between signal measurements.

When the scan procedure is initiated, the MR system sets up a matrix of voxels of size $(L_f/N_f) \times (L_p/N_p) \times$ (section thickness) in space inside the bore of the magnet. The object to be scanned is located within this voxel matrix, which is fixed in space. The effect of motion is to change the tissue content of voxels as the motion moves anatomical structures through the matrix between or during signal measurements. The change in tissue content of a voxel is reflected as a change in the value of $M(x,y)$, which in turn will change the amplitude of the signal arising from that voxel for successive signal measurements. This effect of motion is most pronounced for voxels located at the interface of regions of different tissue content. Voxels located centrally within a region of homogeneous tissue content will not undergo a significant change in tissue content (if the amplitude of the motion is small compared with the size of the region itself).

Consider the signal arising from a stationary source located in the voxel centered at (x,y). Immediately following a 90° excitation pulse, transverse magnetization

[M(x,y)] will be created in this voxel. The amount of transverse magnetization created within the voxel by each excitation pulse will remain constant over time (Figure 10-1A). This transverse magnetization will rotate around the B_0 field at the resonance frequency (ω_0). This would generate a voltage in the receiver coil that varies in a sinusoidal manner at frequency ω_0 and in phase with the reference signal. If we temporarily ignore the phase- and frequency-encoding gradients, then this voltage will be proportional to the function $M(x,y)\cos(2\pi\omega_0 t)$ (Figure 10-2A). The Fourier transform of this voltage will yield the value $M(x,y)$ at the single frequency ω_0 (Figure 10-3A).

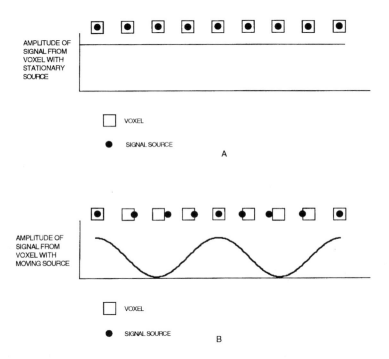

FIGURE 10-1. (A) The amplitude of the signal from a stationary source remains constant over time. (B) As a moving source moves into and out of a voxel, the amplitude of the signal emitted by the voxel varies in a sinusoidal manner over time.

Consider the signal arising from a moving source located in the voxel centered at (x,y). Suppose the motion is sinusoidal in nature at frequency ω_m and that the source moves into and out of the voxel over time (Figure 10-1B). When the source is completely within the voxel at the time of excitation, the transverse magnetization created within the voxel will equal $M(x,y)$. When the source is completely outside of the voxel at the time of excitation, the transverse magnetization created will equal zero. The transverse magnetization following each excitation pulse will then vary in a periodic manner at frequency ω_m. This would generate a voltage in the receiver

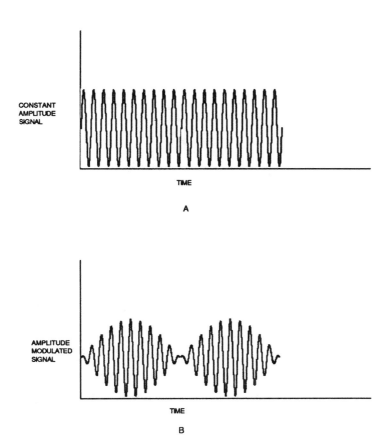

FIGURE 10-2. (A) The signal emitted by a voxel containing a stationary source. (B) The signal emitted by a voxel containing a moving source. The amplitude of the signal changes over time. This is usually referred to as modulation of the signal amplitude.

coil whose amplitude varies in a sinusoidal manner at frequency ω_m (Figure 10-2B) and in phase with the reference signal. Since the amplitude is a periodic function at frequency ω_m, it can be represented by a sum of cosine (and sine) functions at frequencies that are integral multiples of ω_m. The m-th term of the sum (for the cosine functions) will equal $A_m\cos(2\pi m\omega_m t)$. If we again temporarily ignore the phase- and frequency-encoding gradients, then the induced voltage will now be proportional to a function that is a sum of terms of the form $M(x,y)A_m\cos(2\pi m\omega_m t)\cos(2\pi\omega_0 t)$.

What happens when we take the Fourier transform of the above function (Figure 10-3B)? The following identity is needed: $\cos(\omega_1)\cos(\omega_2) = [\cos(\omega_1 + \omega_2) + \cos(\omega_1 - \omega_2)]/2$. That is, the product of two cosine functions at frequencies ω_1 and ω_2 is equal to a sum of two cosine functions at frequencies $(\omega_1 + \omega_2)$ and $(\omega_1 - \omega_2)$.

Therefore, $\cos(2\pi m\omega_m t)\cos(2\pi\omega_0 t) = [\cos(2\pi[\omega_0 + m\omega_m]t) + \cos(2\pi[\omega_0 - m\omega_m]t)]/2$. Note that for m = 0 the product reduces to $\cos(2\pi\omega_0 t)$. The voltage induced in the receiver coil by the moving source will then be equal to the following:

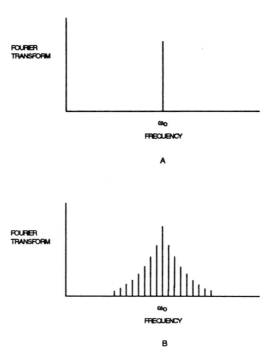

FIGURE 10-3. (A) The Fourier transform of a single cosine function yields a single frequency. (B) The Fourier transform of a sum of cosine functions yields multiple frequencies with varying amplitudes.

$$A_0 M(x,y)\cos(2\pi\omega_0 t) + A_1 M(x,y)[\cos(2\pi[\omega_0 + \omega_m]t) + \cos(2\pi[\omega_0 - \omega_m]t)]/2 + \cdots + \text{etc.}$$

The effect of the motion, then, is to introduce additional frequency components into the voltage.

In the above discussion, we ignored frequency and phase encoding. As discussed in Chapter 8, the frequency-encoding gradient causes the voltage induced by a voxel to vary as a function of time as well as position along the frequency-encoding direction. Likewise, the phase-encoding gradient causes the voltage induced by a voxel to vary as a function of gradient strength as well as position along the phase-encoding direction. As the voltage is sampled, each sample corresponds to a different spatial frequency along both the frequency- and phase-encoding directions. The Fourier transform converts the voltage obtained at these spatial frequencies (k_x and k_y) into signal amplitudes at different locations along the x and y axes.

The effect of the additional temporal frequency components in the induced voltage as a result of the periodic motion of the source is different for the frequency and phase-encoding directions. As noted in Chapter 8, the temporal frequency $m\omega_m$ corresponds to the spatial position $m\omega_m/\gamma G$ along the frequency- encoding direction (x axis). Since phase samples are separated in time by an interval of length TR, the temporal frequency $m\omega_m$ corresponds to a phase change of $m\omega_m TR$ between phase samples ($m\omega_m$ is in units of cycles per second and TR is in unit of seconds so that $m\omega_m$TR is in units of cycles). As noted in Chapter 8, this corresponds to the spatial position $m\omega_m$TR/$\gamma\Delta$Ht along the phase-encoding direction (y axis).

To summarize, then, periodic motion at frequency ω_m will result in additional temporal frequency components in the induced voltage. When a Fourier transform is performed on this voltage, these additional temporal frequency components will be converted into additional sources of signal along the frequency- and phase-encoding directions and will be displayed as ghosts within the MR image. The spacing between ghosts along the frequency-encoding direction is ω_m/γG and along the phase-encoding direction is ω_mTR/$\gamma\Delta$Ht.

With respect to the frequency-encoding direction, γG will be on the order of 1 kHz or more. For respiratory motion or cardiac motion, ω_m will be on the order of 1 Hz or less. Therefore, ω_m/γG will be essentially zero and no ghosts will be visible along the frequency-encoding direction. On the other hand, with respect to the phase-encoding direction, $\gamma\Delta$Ht is on the order of one cycle per centimeter, ω_mTR is on the order of several cycles, and, therefore, ω_mTR/$\gamma\Delta$Ht will be on the order of several centimeter or less. Therefore, motion-induced ghosts are usually visible only along the phase-encoding direction.

The above makes intuitive sense. During each signal measurement, samples are obtained extremely rapidly in the presence of the frequency-encoding gradient (usually on the order of one-tenth of a millisecond between frequency samples). Except for flowing blood, there will be essentially no physiologic motion between frequency samples. On the other hand, the interval of time between signal measurements (made with different strength phase-encoding gradients) is equal to TR. TR is typically on the order of seconds. There will be significant physiologic motion between phase samples. In the presence of this motion, tissues may be in very different locations in the fixed voxel matrix. When the phase-encoding gradient is applied, the tissue acquires a phase that is greater or less than the intended value, because the tissue has moved. The Fourier transform in the phase direction interprets the phase correctly, placing the tissue in a location in the voxel matrix that corresponds to the phase change imposed by the phase-encoding gradient. The location in the image matrix is also incorrect. For this reason, motion-induced ghost artifact is typically only seen along the phase-encoding direction. It is important to remember, however, that motion in any direction (whether along the phase-encoding direction or the frequency-encoding direction, or both) results in phase ghosts (Figure 10-4).

In the discussion above, no mention was made of the direction of motion. In fact, the direction of motion is irrelevant as far as the production of ghosts is concerned. It is simply the periodic change in signal intensity (resulting from motion) that causes the ghosts. The amplitudes of the ghosts arising from a moving structure are directly proportional to the signal intensity of the structure itself. Whatever the signal intensity of the structure of origin, A_m decreases rapidly with increasing values of m. In fact, only the first several ghosts will usually be of sufficient amplitude to be visible on MR images.

Interestingly, phase ghosts can be produced in the absence of any type of motion (Figures 10-5 and 10-6). If the time between excitations of a pulse sequence (i.e., the TR) is made to vary in a periodic manner, then the degree of recovery of

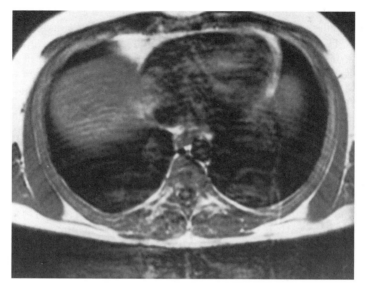

A

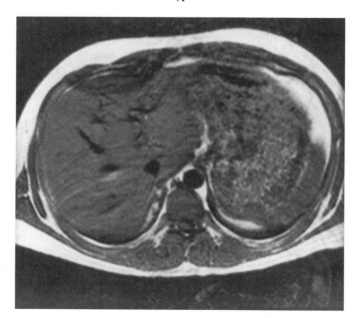

B

FIGURE 10-4 A & B. (A) Axial T1-weighted image through the upper abdomen with the phase direction oriented anteroposterior. Respiratory ghost artifact from the anterior abdominal wall is seen as multiple lines displayed through the image. (B) Image through the midabdomen obtained in the same patient as in (A) shows prominent ghost artifact through the liver.

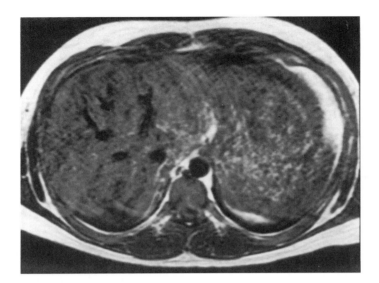

FIGURE 10-4C.   Image obtained at same level as in (B) but with phase oriented from left to right. The lines from ghost artifact are now seen to be in a criss-cross pattern from left to right.

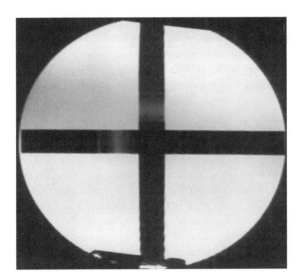

FIGURE 10-5.   Image obtained through stationary phantom with a fixed TR.

longitudinal magnetization between excitations will also vary periodically. This results in a periodic variation of signal intensity and therefore produces ghosts. This would usually occur only with gated sequences, where the time between excitations varies as a function of either the cardiac or respiratory cycle.

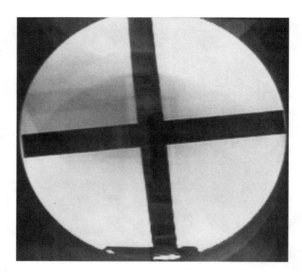

FIGURE 10-6. Image obtained through stationary phantom with a variable TR. Ghost artifact appears identical to that which would occur secondary to motion.

Since ghosts are often superimposed on other tissue within the image, the net signal at the location of a ghost is the sum of the signal from the ghost and the signal from the underlying tissue. If these two signals are in phase, there will be an increase in signal intensity. If these two signals are out of phase, there will be a decrease in the signal intensity (Figures 10-7A–C). This accounts for the seemingly paradoxical areas of low signal that can occur from ghosts that arise from very high signal structures (such as vessels). The phase of the ghost signal is determined by the phase of the motion. In turn, the phase of the motion is independent of the phase of tissue signals.

1.2 RESPIRATORY ORDERED PHASE ENCODING

How can ghost artifact be reduced? Since ghosts arise from periodic motion, if one can eliminate periodic motion, one can eliminate ghosts. The most troublesome ghosts arise from respiratory motion and vascular pulsation and flow variations. There are two techniques commonly used to reduce the ghosts that arise from these types of motion.

Respiratory ordered phase encoding (ROPE) is commonly employed when imaging the abdomen and/or pelvis with conventional spin echo pulse sequences. This technique essentially converts periodic motion into nonperiodic motion with respect to the phase-encoding process. How is this achieved?

A different phase-encoding gradient strength is used for each excitation of an MRI sequence. The number of different phase-encoding gradient strengths is equal to the size of the phase matrix. The difference in strength between successive phase-encoding gradients is a constant (denoted by ΔH in the above discussion). For most

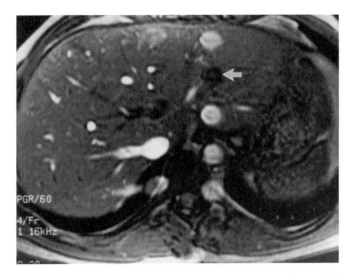

FIGURE 10-7A. Axial gradient echo two-dimensional time of flight (TOF) sequence through the level of the upper abdomen. There is prominent ghost artifact originating from the aorta. Most of the ghosts are of high signal. However, there is a ghost superimposed over the left lobe of the liver that shows low signal (arrow). Low-signal and high-signal ghosts originate from the inferior vena cava (IVC) and hepatic veins.

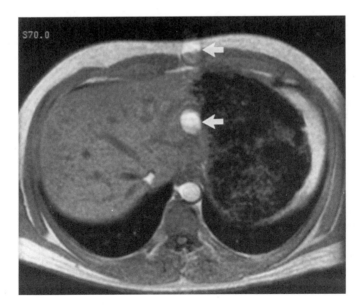

FIGURE 10-7B. Axial T1-weighted image obtained without saturation pulses shows high signal in the aorta and prominent ghost artifact (arrows).

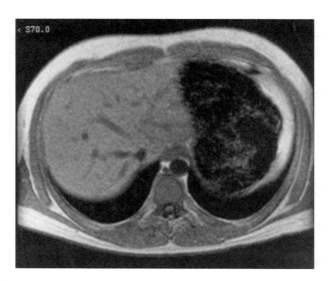

FIGURE 10-7C. Image at identical level as in (B) and with identical parameters except that superior and inferior saturation pulses were used. There is near signal void within the aorta and inferior vena cava and elimination of ghost artifact.

imaging sequences, the phase-encoding gradients are applied in sequential fashion from the strongest negative gradient to the strongest positive gradient. Suppose the size of the phase matrix is 128. Denote the negative-most gradient as $-G_{64}$ and the positive-most gradient as $+G_{64}$.

As a simple example, suppose that TR is equal to one-half the period of the respiratory cycle. In addition, suppose the first excitation is begun at full inspiration. Then the second excitation will occur at full expiration. The third excitation will occur at full inspiration, and so on. Therefore, excitations will alternate on full inspiration and full expiration. If the phase-encoding gradients are applied in sequential fashion (from most negative to most positive), there would be a periodic variation of the signal intensity between successive phase-encoded signal measurements.

On the other hand, suppose the phase-encoding gradients are applied in the order $-G_{64}$, $+G_{64}$, $-G_{63}$, $+G_{63}$, etc. This means that successive negative phase-encoding gradients are all applied at full inspiration and successive positive phase-encoding gradients are all applied at full expiration (Figure 10-8 A and B). This is precisely equivalent to applying the phase-encoding gradients in sequential fashion from the strongest negative gradient to the strongest positive gradient with only a single breath in between. Therefore, by reordering the phase-encoding gradients with respect to the respiratory cycle, we have essentially eliminated periodic motion between successive phase-encoding gradients.

ROPE is implemented by using a hollow tube closed at one end with the other end connected to a pressure transducer. The tube is wrapped around the patient's abdomen or pelvis. The average respiratory rate is determined and the order of application of the phase-encoding gradients is adjusted based on the respiratory cycle

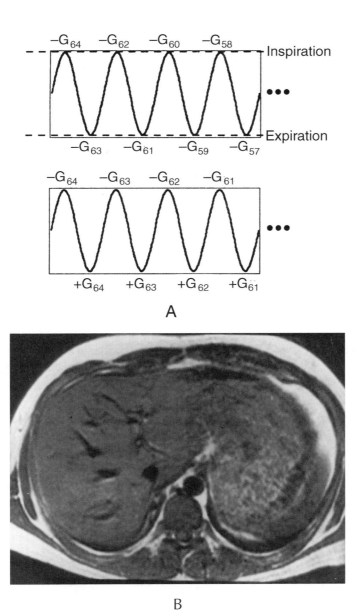

A

B

FIGURE 10-8. (A) The respiratory cycle is represented by a sinusoidal function with full inspiration at the peaks and full expiration at the troughs. If the phase-encoding gradients are applied in sequential fashion from most negative to most positive (upper trace), there will be a periodic variation of the signal intensity from voxels through which structures move. By applying the gradients as shown in the lower trace, it is equivalent to imaging with a single respiratory cycle. (B) Image obtained at same level as that in Figure 10-4B and C but with respiratory compensation. There is near complete elimination of respiratory ghost artifact.

to reduce the effective periodic motion between successive phase-encoding gradients. It is usually more complicated than the simple example given above.

1.3   RESPIRATORY/CARDIAC TRIGGERING

For most MRI sequences, a fixed value of TR is chosen based upon the image contrast desired. This value is not necessarily related in any way to the time between respiratory cycles and/or cardiac cycles. However, the data acquisition can be acquired such that the spacing between excitations is chosen to equal an integral multiple of either the respiratory or cardiac cycle. This will essentially eliminate motion between excitations. As long as the interval between excitations is relatively constant (in this sense, relatively means that the TR is not that variable), ghosts can be reduced or eliminated. Gating of data acquisitions will be discussed later in this chapter.

2   ALIASING (WRAPAROUND ARTIFACT)

A problem that arises as a result of the signal measurement process and Fourier transformation is aliasing. Aliasing (or wraparound) in MR images is the appearance of parts of anatomical structures where they do not belong. A familiar MRI example is the appearance of the nose at the back of the head in a sagittal image of the head (Figure 10-9). An even more common example is the appearance of wagon wheels in western movies. Sometimes the wheels appear to be rotating backwards when the wagon is moving forward. We will review the ADC process, signal sampling, and the Fourier transformation in order to understand the origin of aliasing and methods to eliminate it.

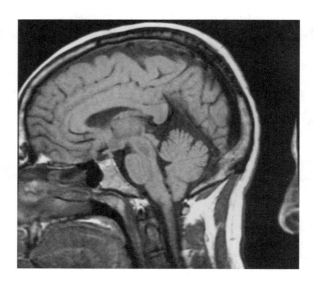

FIGURE 10-9.   Sagittal image through the head with phase oriented anterior to posterior shows wraparound of the nose (located outside of the FOV anteriorly) to a position posterior to the head.

The MR signal is generated by transverse magnetization rotating in the xy plane. This can be represented by a rotating vector (V_1). Suppose that V_1 is initially oriented along the positive y axis and suppose that it rotates **clockwise**. Suppose that after a period of time Δt, V_1 has rotated 270° clockwise. At this point in time V_1 will be oriented along the negative x axis. On the other hand, suppose a second vector (V_2) is initially oriented along the positive y axis and suppose that it rotates **counterclockwise** at one-third the rate of V_1. After the period of time Δt, V_2 will also be oriented along the negative x axis. In general, a clockwise rotation of $\vartheta°$ is indistinguishable from a counterclockwise rotation of $(360 - \vartheta)°$, for $180° < \vartheta° < 360°$ (Figure 10-10).

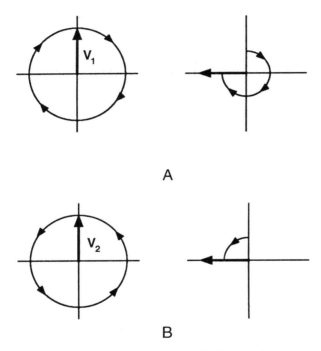

FIGURE 10-10. (A) A vector rotating clockwise initially located along the positive y axis undergoes a positive 270° rotation. (B) A vector rotating counterclockwise initially located along the positive y axis undergoes a negative 90° rotation. Both vectors rotate onto the negative x axis, and the result of the clockwise 270° rotation is indistinguishable from the counterclockwise 90° rotation.

According to the Nyquist theorem, in order to accurately characterize the rate of rotation of a vector, the vector position must be sampled at intervals of less than 180° rotations. This corresponds to intervals of at most one half cycle (since 180° corresponds to a half cycle).

The MR signal is measured in the presence of the frequency- encoding gradient. This causes the signal to consist of many frequency components. As previously described, the frequency-encoding gradient is a linear gradient that causes the local field strength at the point (x,y) to differ from B_0 by Gx, where G is the amplitude of the gradient. G is in units of Gauss per centimeter. Transverse magnetization at the point (x,y) will rotate at a frequency that differs from the resonance frequency (ω_0) by γGx. At x = 0, transverse magnetization will rotate at the resonance frequency. For positive values of x, transverse magnetization will rotate at frequencies greater than ω_0, and for negative values of x, transverse magnetization will rotate at frequencies less than ω_0.

By definition, the FOV of an MR image is the physical length (along both the frequency- and phase-encoding directions) over which the image extends. The FOV may not include all tissue within an excited plane or section, depending on the size of the object being imaged. For example, when an axial section is obtained, the section select gradient is applied along the z direction so that all tissue having z coordinates between certain values will be excited. As a result, all structures within the magnet at the specified axial location will be excited. In most applications, the image will be square so that a single value for the FOV is specified. The frequency-encoding gradient changes the precessional frequency across the FOV. The bandwidth of frequencies contained in the FOV is equal to the difference between the highest and lowest frequencies at either end of the FOV.

Suppose the strength of the frequency- encoding gradient is such that the frequency at one end of the FOV is (ω_0 – 16 kHz) and the frequency at the other end is (ω_0 + 16 kHz). Voxels located between the ends of the FOV along the frequency-encoding direction will produce signal at frequencies between these values. Under this circumstance, the bandwidth across the FOV is usually specified as ±16 kHz. For many imaging systems ±16 kHz is the default value of the bandwidth (unless specifically changed by the user). When the FOV is chosen, the imaging system automatically adjusts the strength of the frequency-encoding gradient so that the bandwidth across the chosen FOV is equal to ±16 kHz. The minimum FOV is therefore dependent upon the maximum gradient strength of the system.

When an excitation pulse is applied, all tissue within a given section is excited, even those portions of the section outside of the FOV (Figure 10-11). Those portions of the sample within the excited section that are outside of the FOV, will precess at frequencies greater than (ω_0 + 16 kHz) at one end of the FOV and at frequencies less than (ω_0 – 16 kHz) at the other end.

According to the Nyquist theorem, when performing an ADC, the sampling frequency for digitization must be at least twice the frequency of the highest frequency component present in the signal. The sampling frequency is usually chosen such that it equals exactly twice the highest frequency component. For the default bandwidth of ±16 kHz, the sampling frequency would then be chosen to equal 32 kHz. The total number of frequency samples is equal to the size of the frequency matrix. At a sampling rate of 32 kHz (32,000 samples per second, which equals 32 samples per millisecond), the sampling time will equal 256/32 = 8 ms.

In MRI, the received signal contains frequencies in the megahertz range (where 1 MHz = one million cycles per second) since the resonance frequency is 63.87 MHz. If the received signal itself was digitized, this would require a sampling frequency in the 100-MHz range, which is not practical. The ADCs in most MRI

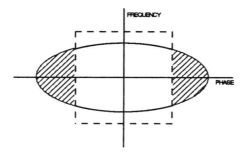

FIGURE 10-11. An elliptical object is shown with its long axis oriented along the phase-encoding direction. The FOV is indicated by the dashed square. Portions of the object that extend beyond the FOV are cross-hatched.

systems actually use a process called heterodyning to digitize the signal. Through this process, the resonance frequency is actually subtracted from the frequencies of the received signal. The resulting (difference) signal then contains frequencies in the kilohertz range and it is this signal that is actually sampled and digitized.

How is this process of subtracting the resonance frequency from the received signal actually performed? Suppose the MR signal contains the single frequency component ω, where $\omega = \omega_0 + \Delta\omega$, and where $|\Delta\omega|$ is very small compared with ω_0 (the symbol $|\ |$ denotes absolute value). ω_0 is the "center frequency," which is carefully determined for each scan sequence. Form the product $P = \cos(\omega t)\cos(\omega_0 t)$. As discussed above, the product of two cosine functions at frequencies ω and ω_0 is equal to $(1/2)[\cos(\omega + \omega_0)t + \cos(\omega - \omega_0)t]$, and since $\omega - \omega_0 = \Delta\omega$, this will equal $(1/2)[\cos(\omega + \omega_0)t + \cos(\Delta\omega)t]$.

Then P will equal the sum of a very-high-frequency component $[\cos(\omega + \omega_0)t]$ and a much lower frequency component $[\cos(\Delta\omega)t]$ (Figure 10-12). The period of the high-frequency component is $1/(\omega + \omega_0)$. The period of the low-frequency component is $1/(\Delta\omega)$. Since $\Delta\omega$ is very small compared to $\omega + \omega_0$, $1/(\Delta\omega)$ will greatly exceed $1/(\omega + \omega_0)$. For example, suppose $\Delta\omega = 100$ Hz so that $\omega = 63.87$ MHz + 100 Hz. Then $1/(\omega + \omega_0) < 10^{-8}$ and $1/(\Delta\omega) = 0.01$. This means that over a given interval of time, the function $\cos(\omega + \omega_0)t$ will go through many more cycles than the function $\cos(\Delta\omega)t$.

What is the average value of a sinusoidal function over a given interval of time? If the function goes through many cycles over the interval, the average value will approach zero. This results from the fact that a sinusoidal function varies from positive to negative values in a periodic manner. The average value of the sum $[\cos(\omega + \omega_0)t + \cos(\Delta\omega)t]$ over a period of time T is equal to the sum of the average values.

In the example above, choose $T = 0.01/2 = 0.005$. The function $\cos(\Delta\omega)t$ will go through one-half cycle over this time. However, $\cos(\omega + \omega_0)t$ will go through greater than 500,000 cycles over this same time. The average value of $\cos(\omega + \omega_0)t$ will be essentially zero over this interval. Therefore, the average value of the sum over the interval T will equal the average value of the function $\cos(\Delta\omega)t$ alone.

A

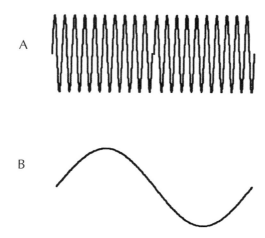

B

FIGURE 10-12. (A) A plot of the high-frequency component, $\cos(\omega + \omega_0)t$. (B) A plot of the low-frequency component, $\cos(\Delta\omega)t$.

If the average value of the above sum is calculated or measured over many consecutive intervals of length T, a series of average values will be generated. These will be the average values of the function $\cos(\Delta\omega)t$. The average value will also vary in a periodic manner at frequency $\Delta\omega$. By performing an ADC and Fourier transform on this series of average values, we can therefore determine the value of $\Delta\omega$. Since ω_0 is known, and $\omega = \omega_0 + \Delta\omega$, we can then determine the value of ω, which is what we wanted to do in the first place. We have, however, accomplished this by sampling at a much lower frequency (namely, $2\Delta\omega = 200$ Hz in the example above).

We have accomplished the determination of ω by sampling the average value of the product of $\cos\omega t$ with a reference signal at the resonance frequency (namely, $\cos\omega_0 t$). The sampling rate required is much lower than would otherwise be required if we sampled $\cos\omega t$ directly. The sampling for this process is identical to an ADC except that we use the average value of a function over a short interval of time rather than instantaneous values of a function at specific points in time. Once the set of discrete values is determined (with either process) the data is handled in an identical manner.

One problem remains. In the above discussion, $\Delta\omega$ may be negative or positive, because the gradient lowers the precession frequency on one side of the FOV, while raising the precession frequency on the other side. So ω may be greater than or less than ω_0 and we would get the same result, because $\cos(\vartheta) = \cos(-\vartheta)$ for all values of ϑ. Therefore, if the signal $\cos\omega t$ is compared only with the reference signal $\cos\omega_0 t$, we would be unable to determine if ω is greater than or less than ω_0. The comparison can detect only the difference in frequency ($\Delta\omega$) between the two signals. In order to determine whether the frequency difference is positive or negative, the signal $\cos\omega t$ is also multiplied by a phase-shifted reference signal, $\cos(\omega_0 t - 90°)$. By choice, the second reference is phase shifted by $-90°$. We could have just as easily used a phase shift of $+90°$ for the second reference. It is important only that we know which phase shift is chosen. Why does this work?

Suppose a vector (V) rotates clockwise at frequency ω. Suppose a second vector (V_{ref}) rotates at frequency ω_0. Suppose that at time t = 0 both vectors are aligned along the positive y axis. As time goes on, the vectors will begin to separate. If one measures the separation over time, it will vary in a sinusoidal manner at a frequency equal to $|\omega - \omega_0|$. It would be impossible to determine which vector rotates more rapidly. The period of the difference frequency is $1/(|\omega - \omega_0|)$. Therefore, the vectors will be 180° out of phase at time t = $1/2(|\omega - \omega_0|)$. Suppose that vector V is along the positive x axis at time t = $1/2(|\omega - \omega_0|)$ and vector V_{ref} is along the negative x axis at this time.

Repeat the experiment with the phase of V_{ref} shifted backward by 90° so that at time t = 0 V_{ref} is along the negative x axis and V (as it was before) is along the positive y axis. The relative position of the two vectors at time t = $1/2(|\omega - \omega_0|)$ is now different. If V_{ref} is rotating more rapidly, then it will be 90° ahead in phase at this time. In this case, at time t = $1/2(|\omega - \omega_0|)$, V will be along the positive x axis and V_{ref} will be along the negative y axis (Figure 10-13 B). On the other hand, if V_{ref} is rotating more slowly it will be 90° behind in phase at this time. In this case, at time t = $1/2(|\omega - \omega_0|)$, V will be along the positive x axis and V_{ref} will be along the positive y axis (Figure 10-13 C). Therefore, the position of the vectors is uniquely determined by taking two measurements with one of the reference vectors shifted in phase by a known amount (Figure 10-13).

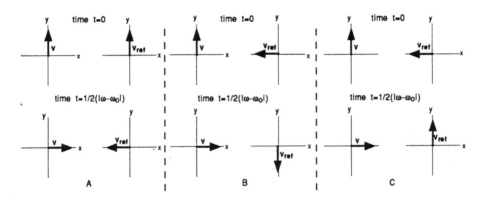

FIGURE 10-13. (A) At time t = 0, V and V_{ref} are both oriented along the positive y axis. At time t = $1/2|\omega - \omega_0|$, the two vectors are 180° out of phase with V along the positive x axis and V_{ref} along the negative x axis. (B) and (C): The experiment is repeated such that at time t = 0, V_{ref} is phase shifted by –90° so that it is oriented along the negative x axis. If V_{ref} is rotating more rapidly than V, it will now be oriented along the negative y axis (as in B). If V_{ref} is rotating more slowly than V, it will now be oriented along the positive y axis (as in C).

When MRI is performed, the received signal is fed into two separate channels for analysis. In one channel it is compared with the reference $\cos\omega_0 t$, and in the second channel it is compared to the reference $\cos(\omega_0 t - 90°)$. Note that $\cos(\omega_0 t - 90°) = \sin\omega_0 t$. By comparing the phase shift of the signals in the two separate channels, we can determine whether the signal $\cos\omega t$ is of higher or lower frequency than the reference signal $\cos\omega_0 t$.

The signals in each channel are digitized and Fourier transformed separately. In this way, the received signal is broken into two component signals that are 90° out of phase. The signals from the two channels are said to be in **quadrature**. The component in phase with the reference $\cos\omega_0 t$ is sometimes referred to as the **real image**, and the component 90° out of phase with this reference (i.e., in phase with the reference $\sin\omega_0 t$) is sometimes referred to as the **imaginary image**. The terms real and imaginary are mathematical only.

Denote the signal in the channel using the reference $\cos\omega_0 t$ by R (for real). Denote the signal in the channel using the reference $\sin\omega_0 t$ by I (for imaginary). As noted above, the signals in each of these channels is separately Fourier transformed. The individual signal in each channel can be used to reconstruct an image. However, the S/N is maximized by reconstructing a so called **magnitude image** (denoted by M). The signal intensity in each pixel of the magnitude image is equal to the square root of the sum of the squares of the pixel intensities in the real and imaginary images. That is, $M = \sqrt{(R^2 + I^2)}$.

The above process using two separate channels in comparing the received signal to a reference signal is referred to as **phase-sensitive detection**, or **quadrature detection**. The use of the term quadrature here is in no way related to a quadrature coil. That is, a quadrature coil is not required for quadrature detection. The above signal comparison process uses a single signal as an input (whether from a single linear coil or the combined signals from a quadrature coil) fed into two separate receiver channels for analysis.

What does all this have to do with aliasing? Aliasing occurs when the MR signal is not sampled rapidly enough. Consider first frequency aliasing. Suppose the size of the FOV along the frequency-encoding direction is 2L. This means that (along the x axis) the FOV extends from x = –L to x = L. If the signal sampling frequency is 32 kHz, then the frequency-encoding gradient strength will be such that the frequency of the signal emitted from the voxel with spatial coordinates (x,y) will equal $\omega_0 + 16(x/L)$ kHz. For example, when x = L, the emitted signal will have frequency ($\omega_0 + 16$ kHz) and when x = –L, the emitted signal will have frequency ($\omega_0 - 16$ kHz). If a portion of an object extends beyond the physical dimensions of the FOV along the frequency-encoding direction (Figure 10-14), then the frequency of its signal will differ from the resonance frequency by more than 16 kHz.

For example, suppose a voxel is located at x coordinate +3L/2. This voxel will emit signal at 24 kHz above the resonance frequency. This signal will advance through 3/4 of a positive cycle (24/32) between frequency samples. However, 3/4 of a positive cycle is indistinguishable from 1/4 of a negative cycle (Figure 10-10). The voxel with x coordinate –L/2 will advance through 1/4 of a negative cycle between frequency samples. Therefore, the signal from the voxel with x coordinate +3L/2 will be misregistered at x coordinate –L/2. This positional misregistration is commonly referred to as wraparound or aliasing artifact. A portion of an object that extends beyond the high-frequency side of the FOV is misregistered (or wrapped around) to the low-frequency side, and vice versa (Figure 10-15).

Two methods are used to prevent frequency aliasing. The simplest is to filter the received signal. The receiver uses a bandpass filter, which attenuates all frequencies outside of a desired range. In this way, frequencies outside of the range ($\omega_0 \pm 16$ kHz)

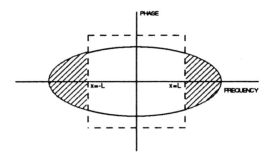

FIGURE 10-14. An oval object is oriented as shown. The FOV is indicated by the dashed square.

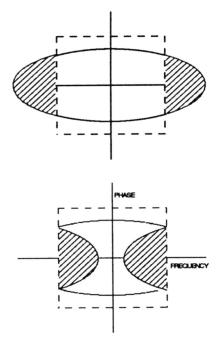

FIGURE 10-15. (A) The field of view is shown by the dashed square. Portions of the object that extend beyond the confines of the FOV along the frequency-encoding direction are cross-hatched. (B) In the image, the cross-hatched regions are misregistered (or wrapped) onto opposite ends of the FOV.

can be filtered out of the received signal. A bandpass filter is routinely used by most imaging systems.

A second method that can be used to avoid frequency aliasing is to increase the sampling rate. Instead of using a sampling rate of 32 kHz, the machine oversamples using a sampling frequency of 64 kHz. This allows accurate determination of frequencies in the range $\omega_0 \pm 32$ kHz. This essentially doubles the effective size of the FOV along the frequency-encoding direction without changing the strength of the frequency-encoding gradient. The signal emitted from voxels with x coordinate up to ±2L can now be accurately sampled. Most MRI systems employ oversampling and frequency filtering for all scans.

As previously noted, when the signal is sampled in the presence of the frequency-encoding gradient, the total number of samples is equal to the size of the frequency matrix. At a sampling rate of 32 kHz, the sampling time for 256 samples will be 8 ms. If the sampling rate is increased to 64 kHz, the sampling time for 256 samples will be 4 ms. In order to maintain a constant S/N, when the sampling rate is increased to 64 kHz, 512 samples are actually obtained so that the sampling time remains constant at 8 ms. Recall that S/N is directly proportional to the sampling time (T_S).

What about aliasing along the phase-encoding direction? If the size of the FOV is 2L along the phase-encoding direction (y axis), then the FOV extends from y = –L to y = L. Position along the phase-encoding direction is determined by the incremental phase change between phase samples. Just as with frequency sampling, according to the Nyquist theorem, the signal must be sampled along the phase-encoding direction such that there is a phase change of at most plus or minus one-half cycle between phase samples. As a function of position along the y axis, the incremental phase change between phase-encoding gradients will therefore equal (1/2)(y/L) cycles. Just as with the frequency-encoding gradient, the largest incremental phase change occurs at the ends of the FOV. If a portion of an object extends beyond the physical dimensions of the FOV along the phase-encoding direction, then it will undergo a phase change of greater than one-half cycle between phase samples.

For example, suppose a voxel is located at y coordinate +3L/2. This voxel will emit signal that undergoes an incremental phase change of 3/4 of a positive cycle between phase samples. However, 3/4 of a positive cycle is indistinguishable from 1/4 of a negative cycle. The voxel with y coordinate –L/2 will undergo an incremental phase change of 1/4 of a negative cycle between phase samples. Therefore, the signal from the voxel with y coordinate +3L/2 will be misregistered at y coordinate –L/2. This positional misregistration is identical to that seen along the frequency-encoding direction (Figure 10-16).

Unlike frequency, there is no way of filtering out unwanted phase changes. The only way to avoid aliasing along the phase-encoding direction is to increase the size of the effective FOV. When an FOV is specified along the phase-encoding direction, the phase-encoding gradient strength increment is adjusted such that voxels located at the ends of the specified FOV undergo a phase change of one-half cycle between phase samples. The larger the size of the FOV, the smaller the increment that is used.

Voxel size along the phase-encoding direction is equal to the FOV divided by the phase matrix size. Therefore, if, for example, the FOV along the phase-encoding direction is doubled and the matrix size remains the same, then voxel size along the phase-encoding direction will also double (which reduces resolution by half). To avoid phase aliasing without losing resolution, the phase FOV and the phase matrix

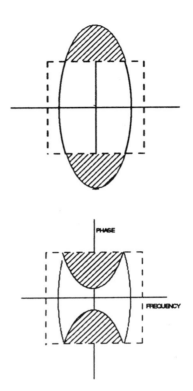

FIGURE 10-16.   Same as Figure 10-15 but with wraparound along the phase-encoding direction.

size can both be doubled. By itself, this would result in a doubling of the scan time (since scan time is directly proportional to the size of the phase matrix).

In order to maintain scan time constant (when doubling the phase matrix) , NSA can be halved (since scan time is directly proportional to the NSA). This is the scheme used on most imaging systems to reduce phase wraparound without changing resolution or imaging time. It is important to note, however, that even this technique will avoid phase wraparound only over a distance equal to twice the chosen FOV. If an FOV of 2L is chosen, even if we double the FOV to 4L, this still means that any portion of anatomy with a y coordinate greater than 2L or less than –2L will undergo wraparound.

Phase wraparound is always more of a problem than frequency wraparound because there is no way of filtering phase. In general, whatever body part is being imaged, on most imaging systems the scanner will (unless instructed otherwise) automatically choose the phase direction along the shortest axis of the anatomy ordinarily imaged in a given coil. Frequency is chosen along the longest such dimension. These are referred to as the default directions.

3   SATURATION PULSES

Depending upon flow velocity and direction, blood vessels will have variable signal intensity on MR images. When intravascular signal is present, it can be problematic because it can give rise to ghost artifact. Vascular ghost artifact arises in two ways. As vessels expand and contract they move through adjacent voxels. This expansion and contraction is periodic with the cardiac cycle. As with respiratory motion, this causes a periodic amplitude modulation of the signal in voxels located adjacent to the vessel and gives rise to phase ghosts (Figure 10-7A).

In addition to the actual motion of the vessel walls, flow velocity varies with the cardiac cycle. Unless an acquisition is gated to the cardiac cycle, this will result in different signal intensities within the vessel at different times of the cardiac cycle. This can result in a periodic variation of the signal intensity of voxels within the lumen of the vessel and can also give rise to phase ghosts.

What determines intravascular signal? When using spin echo pulse sequences, a 180° section selective pulse is applied at time TE/2 following each section selective 90° pulse. All stationary structures will be exposed to both excitation pulses and will emit signal. However, suppose that the flow within a blood vessel is such that the blood excited by the 90° pulse moves out of the section prior to the 180° pulse. Since the 180° pulse is section selective, it will not excite blood that has moved out of the section. In the same manner, the new blood that has flowed into the section will not have been excited by the 90° pulse. As a result, the vessel will appear as a signal void on the MR image. This effect is usually referred to as a **flow-related signal loss**.

On the other hand, suppose that the flow velocity within a vessel is such that the blood excited by the 90° pulse remains within the section at the time of the 180° pulse. In addition, suppose that blood flows out of the section between 90° pulses. Under this circumstance, new blood protons will move into the section between 90° pulses and will remain in the section long enough to be excited by the 180° pulse and emit signal. The blood protons moving into the section between 90° pulses have not been previously excited. This is equivalent to complete recovery of longitudinal magnetization between 90° pulses. This will maximize the signal they emit. This effect is usually referred to as a **flow-related enhancement**.

Consider the following example. For a section of tissue 1 cm thick, in order to have a signal void, the flow velocity must exceed (1 cm)/(TE/2). If TE = 10 ms, then TE/2 = 5 ms and the flow must exceed 1cm/5 ms (= 200 cm/s) to have a signal void. If TE = 20 ms the flow must exceed 100 cm/s to have a signal void. If TE = 80 ms, the flow must exceed 25 cm/s to have signal void. For 5-mm-thick sections these velocities are halved. Therefore, on T1- and proton density–weighted images (which will typically have a TE of 10–20 ms), even arterial flow will rarely result in a complete signal void. On T2-weighted images, most large arteries will have a signal void. Venous flow velocities virtually never result in a signal void on T1-, T2-, or proton density–weighted images.

Both flow-related enhancement and flow-related signal loss are dependent upon the direction of flow with respect to the plane of section. When flow is perpendicular to the plane of section, these effects will be maximal (although which effect predominates is dependent on actual flow velocities). When the flow direction is predominantly within the plane of section, the situation is different. Most (if not all) of the protons within such vessels will remain in the section between the 90° and the 180° pulses. Some fresh protons will enter the section between 90° pulses (i.e., during the TR interval). However, the flowing protons will be moving in the section during application of the frequency- and phase-encoding gradients. Motion during gradient application causes dephasing and therefore signal loss. This dephasing is sufficient to result in signal void for most in-plane vascular flow (especially along the frequency-encoding direction, which has the strongest gradient).

Most MRI sequences acquire the data from many sections during each TR interval. The "stack" of sequential sections can be thought of as an imaging volume. To reduce signal in vascular structures with flow perpendicular to the plane of section, 90° excitation pulses can be applied above and below the imaging volume immediately prior to each sequence of 90° excitation pulses. These are referred to as saturation pulses. The tissue excited by the **saturation pulses**, including the vessels they contain, will acquire transverse magnetization. At the same time, they will have complete loss of longitudinal magnetization.

Immediately following application of the saturation pulses (and before the imaging sequence begins for the first section of the volume), a gradient is applied that causes complete dephasing of the transverse magnetization created by the saturation pulse. This is referred to as a **spoiler gradient**. This causes the blood flowing into the imaging volume to have no net longitudinal magnetization and no net transverse magnetization. Such tissue is said to be saturated, so that when it receives an additional 90° excitation pulse (once it is within the sections of the imaging volume) it emits no signal because it has zero longitudinal magnetization. This is obviously most effective for those sections located at either end of the imaging volume.

Saturation pulses are routinely used to reduce vascular signal when using conventional spin echo pulse sequences (Figures 10-7B and C). However, saturation pulses are often unable to completely eliminate vascular signal and the resultant ghost artifact. The penalty for using saturation pulses is that it takes time to turn the gradients and the pulses on and off. This can slightly reduce the total number of sections that can be acquired for a given TR.

Saturation pulses can also be placed within the imaging FOV. There are several circumstances under which this is useful. For example, when imaging the splenic vein, flow direction can be determined by using saturation pulses within the FOV. On an axial section, the portal vein would course from left to right. A saturation pulse can be placed through the portal vein perpendicular to its course. A small amount of signal will be seen within the edge of the saturation pulse on the in-flow side of the portal vein (Figure 10-17). A second example of using saturation pulses within the FOV is to suppress the signal from subcutaneous fat in the anterior abdominal wall when imaging the abdomen. This can significantly reduce ghost artifact.

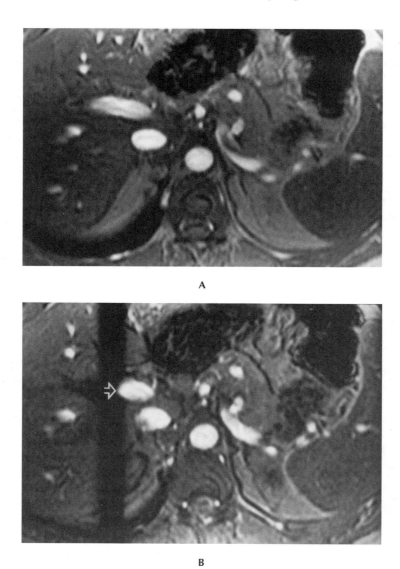

A

B

FIGURE 10-17. In (A), an axial two-dimensional TOF image is obtained at the level of the main portal vein (which shows high signal). In (B), a saturation pulse was placed within the FOV perpendicular to the portal vein. Some high signal extends into the left side of the portal vein (arrow), indicating that flow is from left to right (i.e., toward the liver).

4   FLOW COMPENSATION (GRADIENT MOMENT NULLING)

In some circumstances and with some pulse sequences, it is desirable to maintain intravascular signal. For example, when performing MR angiographic sequences, saturation pulses are disadvantageous. However, when saturation pulses are not used, intravascular signal can result in severe phase ghost artifact (Figure 10-7). As noted in the prior section, this ghost artifact will arise from two separate mechanisms: physical pulsation (i.e., motion) of the vessel wall and variability of vessel flow (due to the cardiac cycle).

What about cerebrospinal fluid (CSF) flow? CSF flow is slow and multidirectional. When CSF flow is predominantly perpendicular to the plane of section, it is too slow to result in signal void. Saturation pulses will be ineffective due to both the slow flow velocity and the multidirectional nature of the flow. Unlike in-plane vascular flow, in-plane CSF flow is usually not of sufficient magnitude to result in signal void from dephasing. Instead, the variability of CSF flow from one excitation to the next will result in a periodic variation of signal intensity and ghost artifact. CSF-induced phase ghosts will be most severe on T2-weighted images where CSF has extremely high signal compared to other structures.

There is an alternative to saturation pulses that can be used to reduce ghost artifact from flowing blood as well as from CSF. This technique is referred to as **flow compensation** (or **gradient moment nulling**). Flow compensation can eliminate dephasing from constant velocity flow along the section select and frequency encoding directions. By eliminating dephasing from constant velocity motion, there will be much less amplitude modulation of the MR signal (from either flowing blood or CSF) and this will reduce or even eliminate ghost artifact. Flow compensation is also used in vascular imaging to increase intravascular signal.

Flow compensation works by applying additional lobes to both the frequency-encoding and section select gradients. These additional lobes can eliminate dephasing from **constant velocity motion**. Any acceleration or higher order pulsatile motion cannot be compensated without using more complex gradients. A penalty for using flow compensation is that it increases the minimum value of TE, because it takes more time to apply the frequency-encoding and section select gradients when they consist of multiple lobes.

How does flow compensation work? When any gradient is applied, it will induce phase changes (in stationary structures) that are directly proportional to the strength of the gradient and the time of application (Figure 10-18). However, if a structure moves while the gradient is being applied, it will experience a variable gradient strength and will therefore be affected in a more complex manner. In the presence of a linear gradient, the phase change induced in protons that undergo constant velocity motion along the gradient direction is directly proportional to gradient strength and velocity of flow and is proportional to the square of the time of gradient application.

This can be seen as follows. Suppose a linear gradient is applied along the x axis (frequency-encoding direction) such that the gradient strength at position x is Gx. The gradient strength is zero at the origin (x = 0). Now the phase change ($\Delta\phi$) induced by a constant gradient is equal to the product of the gradient strength (Gx), the time the gradient is on (t'), and the gyromagnetic ratio (γ). Therefore, the phase change for a stationary proton at position x is equal to $\gamma Gxt'$.

Suppose a proton starts at position x at time t' = 0, at which time the gradient is turned on, and that it moves along the gradient direction with constant velocity v. Then the position of this proton at time t' = t is x + vt. The gradient experienced

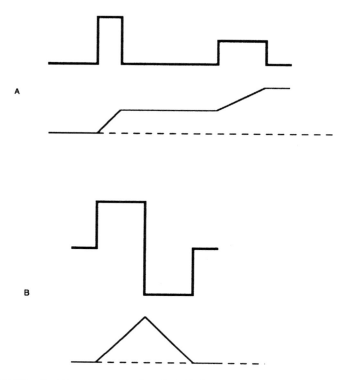

FIGURE 10-18. In (A), a strong gradient is initially turned on for a short time. The phase change is represented by the graph below the gradient. A second gradient of half the strength of the first is then turned on for twice the length of time. The total phase change induced by both gradients is the same. In (B), a bilobed "balanced" gradient is used. The phase change induced by the first half (or first lobe) of the gradient is exactly canceled (or balanced) by the second lobe. The net phase change is zero. Both (A) and (B) assume stationary protons.

by this proton at time t, therefore, is $G(x + vt)$. Over a very short time interval from t to $(t + \Delta t)$, the gradient will be essentially constant, with value $G(x + vt)$, and the phase will change by an amount $\gamma G(x + vt)\Delta t$. In order to determine the total phase change, one need only sum these individual phase changes from $t' = 0$ to $t' = t$. This is equivalent to an integration with respect to t', such that the total phase change is equal to $\gamma Gxt + (1/2)\gamma Gvt^2$. To simplify the discussion below, assume that the proton starts at the origin where $x = 0$. This eliminates the first term of the preceding expression.

During application of the gradient, the proton will move from point $x = 0$ to point $x = vt$. Suppose a gradient is turned on at strength $-G$ as the proton moves from $x = 0$ to $x = vt/4$, at strength $+G$ from $x = vt/4$ to $x = 3vt/4$, and at strength $-G$ from $x = 3vt/4$ to vt. Denote these intervals as 1, 2, and 3, respectively. The magnitude of the phase change over interval 1 is $\gamma Gvt^2/32$. The magnitude of the phase change over interval 2 is $8\gamma Gvt^2/32$. The magnitude of the phase change over interval 3 is $7\gamma Gvt^2/32$. The magnitude of the total phase change over intervals 1 and 3, therefore, is equal to $8\gamma Gvt^2/32$. Since the gradient over interval 2 is positive, and the gradient over intervals 1 and 3 is negative, the total phase change induced by such a gradient for a proton moving at constant velocity is **zero** (Figure 10-19A).

The above calculations use the fact that the phase change over an interval from t to t + k is given by $(1/2)\gamma Gv(t + k)^2 - (1/2)\gamma Gvt^2 = (1/2)\gamma Gv[(t + k)^2 - t^2]$, provided that the gradient is of constant direction over this time. It is obvious that for stationary protons (v = 0), such a gradient (which is balanced) also will induce a phase change of zero.

When the flow compensation option is chosen on MRI systems, just such a trilobed gradient as described above may be used along either or both the section select and frequency-encoding directions, so that there is no gradient-induced phase change for protons moving with constant velocity. This results in increased signal within blood vessels as well as reduction of phase ghost artifact (Figure 10-19 B).

4.1 EVEN ECHO REPHASING

The standard frequency-encoding gradient for a (single echo) spin echo imaging sequence is bilobed. The first lobe is applied immediately after the 90° pulse and the second lobe is applied during the signal measurement. Denote the first lobe as L_1 and the second lobe as L_2. Both lobes are of the same strength (G) and polarity, with L_2 being applied twice as long as L_1. The time of application of L_2 is equal to T_s, the sampling time. If the 90° pulse is applied at time t = 0 and the center of the echo is measured at TE after the 90° pulse, then L_1 is applied from t = 0 to t = $T_s/2$, and L_2 is applied from t = (TE − $T_s/2$) to t = (TE + $T_s/2$).

At the center of L_2, the net phase change for stationary spins will be zero because the phase changes induced by L_1 are exactly canceled at the center of L_2. As noted in the section on flow compensation, the phase change experienced by a proton moving at velocity v over an interval from t to t + k is given by $(1/2)\gamma Gv[(t + k)^2 - t^2]$. Therefore, at the center of L_2, the net phase change for spins moving at constant velocity v will be given by $-(1/2)\gamma Gv(T_s/2)^2 + (1/2)\gamma Gv[TE^2 - (TE - T_s/2)^2]$. The first term is the phase change induced by L_1, and the second term is the phase change induced by the first half of L_2. Note the negative sign in front of the first term, which results from the fact that a 180° pulse is applied after L_1, which reverses the polarity of the induced phase change.

Suppose a two-echo spin echo pulse sequence is performed with echoes acquired at TE and 2TE. This means that 180° pulses are applied at TE/2 and 3TE/2. In order to measure the second echo, a third lobe (L_3) of the frequency-encoding gradient will be applied from t = 2TE − $T_s/2$ to t = 2TE + $T_s/2$.

At the center of L_3, the net phase change for stationary spins will be zero, and the net phase change for spins moving at constant velocity v will equal $(1/2)\gamma Gv(T_s/2)^2 - (1/2)\gamma Gv[(TE + T_s/2)^2 - (TE - T_s/2)^2] + (1/2)\gamma Gv[(2TE)^2 - (2TE - T_s/2)^2]$, which is equal to zero. The first term is the phase change induced by L_1, without a negative sign because two 180° pulses are applied after L_1. The second term is the phase change induced by L_2, with a negative sign because a 180° pulse is applied after L_2. The third term is the phase change induced by the first half of L_3. The pulse diagram is shown in Figure 10-20.

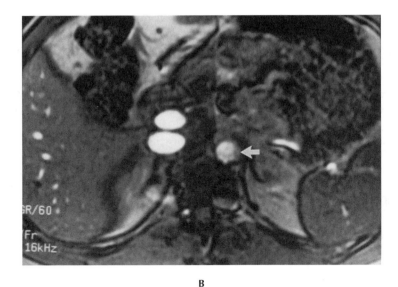

B

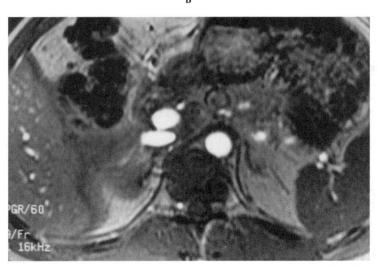

C

FIGURE 10-19 B&C.   Image through the midabdomen obtained without flow compensation shows high signal in the inferior vena cava and portal vein but low signal in the aorta (arrow) with prominent ghost artifact. (C) Image at same level as in (B) obtained with flow compensation. The aorta now shows high signal with minimal ghost artifact.

Due to the intervening application of two 180° pulses, the form of the three lobes of the frequency-encoding gradients is identical to that used for flow compensation. The phase changes induced by L_1 are positive because two 180° pulses are applied after L_1. The phase changes induced by L_2 are negative because a single 180° pulse is applied after L_2. The phase changes induced by L_3 are positive. As

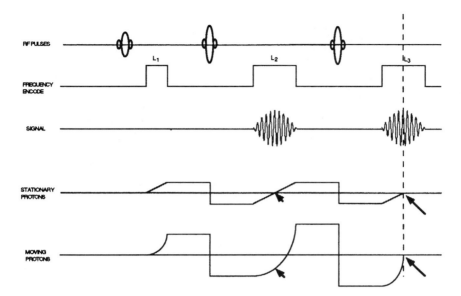

FIGURE 10-20. At the center of the read gradient for the first echo, stationary protons have undergone no net phase change whereas moving protons have undergone a net negative phase change (small arrows). Note that phase changes induced by gradients are reversed after application of a 180° RF pulse. At the center of the read gradient for the second echo, both stationary and moving protons have undergone no net phase change (large arrows).

long as the first and third lobes (of each pair of echoes) are centered around the second lobe, the net phase change induced by protons moving at constant velocity will be zero for the second echo. The same result applies for all even echoes (i.e., fourth echoes, sixth echoes, etc.). This will result in increased intravascular signal for the even echoes of a multiecho acquisition, provided the echoes are evenly spaced. Hence the term **even echo rephasing**.

4.2 VASCULAR POSITIONAL MISREGISTRATION

Flow compensation along the frequency-encoding direction will increase the MR signal in vessels that have flow within the plane of a section. Without flow compensation, such vessels will usually have a signal void unless they have very slow flow. As a result of the increased intravascular signal in vessels with in-plane flow, a different image artifact will arise. This artifact is positional misregistration of vessels. How does this arise?

Consider a blood vessel with flow velocity v, which crosses through an axial section such that it makes an angle of ϑ with the positive x axis. Let the phase-encoding direction be along the y axis and the frequency-encoding direction along the x axis. Let an excitation pulse be applied at time $t = 0$ and a spin echo measured at time $t = TE$. Assume that the phase-encoding gradient is applied over a very short interval of time from $t = 0$ to $t = \tau$ immediately following the excitation pulse.

Consider a proton initially located at position (x_0, y_0). At time $t = \tau$, this same proton will have y coordinate $(y_0 + v\tau\sin\vartheta)$. The factor $\sin\vartheta$ takes into account that the flow is oriented at an angle of $\vartheta°$ with respect to the positive x axis. It can be shown mathematically that the total phase change induced by the phase-encoding gradient for this moving proton will be equal to $\gamma G\tau(y_0 + (v\tau\sin\vartheta)/2)$. The moving proton will therefore undergo the same phase change as a stationary proton with y coordinate given by $(y_0 + (v\tau\sin\vartheta)/2)$. This y coordinate is halfway between the starting and ending coordinates of the moving proton along the y axis during application of the phase-encoding gradient. Therefore, the moving proton will have its position misregistered along the phase direction by an amount equal to half the distance it travels while the phase-encoding gradient is on.

The time over which the phase-encoding gradient is actually on is very short (on the order of a few milliseconds). Therefore, the above positional misregistration along the phase-encoding direction will be minimal.

What about the motion along the frequency-encoding direction between phase and frequency encoding? The time between phase-encoding and the center of frequency-encoding is $\Delta T = TE - \tau$. Over the interval of time ΔT, a proton within the vessel will change its location along the x axis by a distance of $v\Delta T\cos\vartheta$. The factor of $\cos\vartheta$ takes into account that the flow is oriented at an angle of $\vartheta°$ with respect to the positive x axis.

Therefore, the proton initially located at position (x_0, y_0) will have coordinates $(x_0 + v\Delta T\cos\vartheta, y_0 + (v\tau\sin\vartheta)/2)$ in the final image. This holds for each proton within the vessel. This means that the entire vessel will have its position shifted in the final image (Figure 10-21). The shift along the x direction is much greater than the shift along the y direction because $\Delta T \gg \tau$.

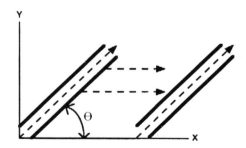

FIGURE 10-21.   A blood vessel is shown as solid lines, with the dashed arrows within the vessels showing the direction of flow. The position of the vessel is shifted along the positive x axis.

Assuming the vessel is relatively straight, only displacements perpendicular to the direction of flow will be apparent. Displacement of the position of a proton from one portion of the vessel along the vessel direction would not be detectable.

5 GATING

Gating (sometimes referred to as triggering) is another method of reducing motion artifacts. This technique was alluded to in the section on reduction of motion-induced ghost artifact. There are two types of gating commonly used: cardiac gating and peripheral gating. With cardiac gating the RF excitation pulses are timed to coincide with the start of systole, using the electrocardiogram (ECG) signal from the patient's heart. With peripheral gating the RF excitation pulses are timed to coincide with the arrival of an increase in oxygen-saturated arterial blood with the peripheral pulse (using a pulse oximeter, commonly attached to a finger). The discussion below refers to cardiac gating, but is applicable to both cardiac and peripheral gating.

With conventional nongated sequences, the time between $90°$ excitation pulses is constant (equal to TR). With gated studies, the time between $90°$ excitation pulses is variable: the timing of the RF excitation pulses depends on the cardiac cycle, specifically on the time between successive QRS peaks in the ECG signal. This interval is called the RR interval. Therefore, the TR is defined (and chosen by the operator) in terms of the RR interval (i.e., TR must equal 1RR, 2RR, 3RR, etc.). As with conventional sequences, many sections are excited during each TR interval.

The QRS peak occurs at the start of systole. The upstroke of the QRS peak in the ECG triggers the imaging sequence. This is usually done by monitoring the voltage across the ECG leads on an oscilloscope or similar display. When imaging is ongoing, gradients are constantly being switched on and off. The gradients induce voltage changes across the ECG lead wires. These voltage changes are superimposed over the ECG trace and can have an amplitude similar to those of the ECG trace itself. In order to prevent gradient-induced voltage changes from triggering the imaging sequence, the imaging system allows triggering only after a specific time, toward the end of the RR interval. This "nonimaging" portion of the RR interval is commonly expressed as a percentage of the RR interval and is often referred to as the trigger window.

If, for example, a patient has an average heart rate of 60 bpm, then the average RR interval is 1000 ms (i.e., 1 s). If a trigger window of 15% is chosen, imaging would be performed for 850 ms after each QRS complex. The last 150 ms of each RR interval (15% of 1000) would be spent waiting for the next QRS. If the patient's heart rate should change such that a QRS complex occurs earlier than 850 ms after the prior QRS complex, it will not trigger the imaging process. The more irregular a patient's heart rate, the larger the trigger window that must be used in order to avoid having beats that will not trigger the imaging sequence.

Because of heart rate variability as well as missed beats, the actual time between $90°$ pulses for a gated sequence will be variable over the course of imaging. If this variability happens to be periodic, it can cause a periodic variation of the signal intensities of structures being imaged. As previously mentioned, this can result in ghost artifact.

Most systems allow the user a choice of the time at which imaging begins following detection of the QRS complex. Since the QRS complex indicates the beginning of systole, when a short delay is used, imaging will begin very close to systole. For most applications, the minimum delay would be used. However, if it is desirable to begin imaging later in the cardiac cycle, a greater delay can be used.

When TR = 2RR or greater, different groups of sections are excited during each RR interval. For example, suppose TR = 2RR and that 10 sections are being imaged. During the first RR interval, sections 1, 3, 5, 7, and 9 are excited, and during the second RR interval sections 2, 4, 6, 8, and 10 can be excited. This is usually referred to as cross-RR imaging and it helps reduce cross excitation between adjacent sections. During a gated acquisition, the image data for each section is obtained at a fixed time following the QRS complex. In the previous example, sections 1 and 2 would be obtained in early systole, sections 3 and 4 slightly later in systole, and so on.

Gated studies also allow the possibility of creating "cine" type images. For cine studies, a single location (or a few locations) is imaged at several phases of the cardiac cycle. For these studies, the TR time is actually much less than a single RR interval. Cine studies are not gated in the prospective manner described above. Cine studies use a gradient echo technique (gradient echo sequences will be discussed in Chapter 11), which allows a very short TR. The ECG tracing is monitored in the computer memory and excitations are obtained in rapid succession at a very short, fixed TR. The computer then retrospectively assigns data to different blocks of time with respect to the cardiac cycle. This allows reconstruction of multiple images, each at the same location but each at a different phase of the cardiac cycle. The images can then be played back in rapid succession in a movie-like manner, which will simulate motion.

Peripheral gating works in an identical manner as cardiac gating. Gating is always used for cardiac imaging to reduce ghost artifact from the moving heart. Gating can also be used to reduce vascular pulsation and CSF pulsation artifact. By gating the study, periodic motion is reduced significantly.

6   HALF FOURIER IMAGING

6.1   FRACTIONAL PHASE DATA ACQUISITION

For most imaging sequences, the phase-encoding gradients are applied in sequential fashion from a maximum negative gradient to a maximum positive gradient (or vice versa). For each positive gradient there is an equal-in-magnitude but opposite-direction negative gradient. The gradients are therefore symmetric about the zero phase-encoded gradient, and the phase-encoded data is symmetric about the zero phase-encoded data.

This means that if the signal that results from application of a positive phase-encoding gradient G is measured, the signal that would result from the phase-encoding gradient –G can be calculated (because these signals will differ only in their phase). In this manner, only half of the phase encoded data is theoretically needed in order to perform a Fourier transform and reconstruct an image. In practice, slightly more than half of the phase encoded data are acquired because the data in the central portion of k space are so important for correct interpretation by the Fourier transform.

The penalty for such an acquisition is reduced S/N because the number of phase samples (N_p) is reduced (even though the size of the phase matrix remains unchanged). The advantage is reduced imaging time, where the total imaging time for such a sequence is equal to TR × (phase matrix size/2) × (NSA). As noted above, the imaging time is actually slightly greater because Np will be slightly greater than (phase matrix size/2).

6.2 FRACTIONAL ECHO

For a spin echo pulse sequence, a 180° pulse is applied at time TE/2 after the 90° pulse. The phase-encoding gradient as well as the first half of the section selective gradient for the 180° pulse must be turned on between the 90° pulse and the 180° pulse. It takes a finite amount of time to turn these gradients on and off. Thus, the minimum time after the 90° pulse at which the 180° pulse can be applied is limited by the time required to turn these gradients on and off. For most imaging systems, this time is at least 3–5 ms.

If a signal sampling rate of 32 kHz is used, the signal measurement process occurs over an 8-ms time interval. The read gradient is therefore turned on 4 ms prior to the echo time (TE) so that the center of the spin echo occurs at the center of the read gradient.

The MR signal cannot be measured until the section selective gradient for the 180° pulse is turned off. Suppose the section selective gradient for the 180° pulse is turned off b milliseconds after the 180° pulse is applied, and that the read gradient is then immediately turned on. The center of the read gradient occurs 4 ms after it is turned on. The center of the echo occurs TE/2 ms after the 180° pulse. Therefore, in order to have the center of the read gradient coincide with the center of the echo, TE/2 = (4 + b) ms. This would make the minimum TE equal to (8 + 2b) milliseconds. Typical values of b on an imaging system are 3–5 ms, making the minimum achievable TE 14–18 ms.

Just as the phase-encoded data are symmetric about the zero phase-encoded gradient, the frequency-encoded data are symmetric about the center of the read gradient. The measured signal can be thought of as consisting of two symmetric halves: one half prior to the center of the read gradient and one half after the center of the read gradient (Figure 10-22). If the first half of the echo is measured, the second half can be calculated and vice versa. Therefore, only a fraction of the echo is required to reconstruct the data from a full echo. In this way, the signal is measured for about half of the time that the frequency-encoding gradient is on. Again, because the central portion of k space data is so important in image production, the fractional echo usually acquires the last 60% of the spin echo.

When using a "fractional echo," the read gradient can be turned on 4 ms earlier than would otherwise be possible (before the section selective gradient for the 180° pulse is even turned off, but after the 180° RF pulse), and signal measurements are performed during the second half of the read gradient (Figure 10-23). In this way, signal measurements are begun almost immediately after the section selective gradient is turned off. The minimum echo time is then reduced by 4 ms and will equal 10–14 ms.

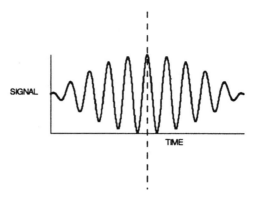

FIGURE 10-22. Representation of MR signal over time. The dashed line is at the center of the read gradient.

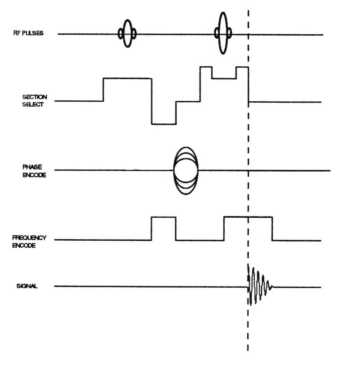

FIGURE 10-23. By only measuring a portion of the echo (i.e., a fraction), the minimum possible TE is obtained. The read gradient is turned on before the last portion of the section select gradient for the 180° pulse is turned off.

The penalty for fractional echo is a reduction of S/N as the sampling time (T_S) is reduced, and the S/N is proportional to the square root of T_S. However, the shorter echo time will result in less signal loss from T2 decay, so that S/N may not actually change significantly. Fractional echo can be used to get truer T1 weighting for conventional spin echo imaging and to get shorter TE values for gradient echo imaging.

6.3 HALF FOURIER ARTIFACT

Ideally, phase-encoded data will be perfectly symmetric about the zero phase-encoding step and frequency-encoded data will be perfectly symmetric about the center of the read gradient. However, due to imperfections in the local magnetic field strength, imperfect RF pulses, small phase shifts in the reference frequency of the quadrature detection circuits, incorrect timing of the read gradient with respect to the spin echo, etc., the data may not always be perfectly symmetric.

For example, suppose that an imperfection in the phase-encoding gradient causes an error in the expected phase shift. Assume the phase-encoding direction is along the y axis. Ideally, if the phase-encoding gradient is of strength +G and is on for time Δt, the phase shift at the point (x,y) will equal $\gamma Gy\Delta t$. Likewise, when the phase-encoding gradient is of strength –G and is on time Δt, the phase shift at the point (x,y) will equal $-\gamma Gy\Delta t$.

Suppose an imperfection (a nonlinearity) in the gradient causes an additional positive phase shift of ϕ at the point (x,y). Then, if the phase-encoding gradient is of strength +G and is on for time Δt, the phase shift at the point (x,y) will equal $\gamma Gy\Delta t + \phi$. Using the assumption of symmetry of data, it would be expected that when the phase-encoding gradient is of strength –G and is on for time Δt, the phase shift at the point (x,y) would equal $-(\gamma Gy\Delta t + \phi)$. The actual phase shift that occurs at the point (x,y) is $-\gamma Gy\Delta t + \phi$. Therefore, the actual phase shift will differ from the expected phase shift. Such errors can result in severe artifacts in the reconstructed image. Spatially dependent phase errors (i.e., phase errors that occur only at certain coordinates) will introduce band-like areas of increased and decreased signal intensity within the image.

When all of the positive and negative phase-encoding gradient steps are collected, these phase errors can be calculated and corrected. However, if only half of the phase-encoded data are collected, these errors cannot be compensated for. Suppose that all of the positive phase-encoding gradient data are collected and a small number of the negative phase-encoding data are also collected. This allows a good estimation of these spatially dependent phase errors and so corrections can be made to the entire data set. It is for this reason that when a fractional phase data acquisition is performed, about 60% of the data is collected in order to allow adequate correction of phase errors. Similarly, when using a fractional echo, about 60% of the full echo is actually measured.

7 CHEMICAL SHIFT SELECTIVE SUPPRESSION

Even when lipid and water protons are exposed to the same external magnetic field, they will precess at slightly different frequencies. This results from slight differences in the chemical environment of the lipid and water protons at the molecular level. Because of these molecular differences, the lipid protons actually experience a slightly smaller local field strength than water protons, even when placed in the same external field. Following excitation, lipid and water protons will therefore emit signal at slightly different frequencies. At a field strength of 1.5 T, the difference in precessional frequency (and therefore the difference in frequency of the emitted signal) is approximately 220 Hz.

The difference in precessional frequency between lipid and water protons can be used to selectively suppress the signal from one or the other. At 1.5 T, water protons precess at 63.87 MHz and lipid protons precess at (63.87 MHz – 220 Hz). Lipid suppression is achieved as follows. A non–section selective narrow bandwidth 90° excitation pulse centered at 63.87 MHz – 220 Hz is applied to the entire imaging volume. The bandwidth of this pulse is on the order of ±100 Hz, so that the maximum frequency component is (63.87 MHz – 120 Hz) and the minimum frequency component is (63.87 MHz – 320 Hz). The maximum frequency component is below the precessional frequency of water protons and, therefore, it will only excite lipid protons.

Immediately following the lipid selective 90° excitation, all of the longitudinal magnetization in lipid containing tissue is converted into transverse magnetization. A strong gradient (referred to as a spoiler gradient) is then turned on, which results in complete loss of transverse magnetization. At this point, lipid-containing tissue has no net transverse or longitudinal magnetization. Immediately following the spoiler gradient the standard spin echo imaging sequence is performed. The lipid protons are now essentially unexcitable because they possess zero longitudinal magnetization. The lipid selective suppression pulse is applied prior to imaging each section in a multisection acquisition (Figure 10-24). In an identical manner, if the narrow bandwidth pulse is centered on the precessional frequency of water protons, the signal from water is selectively suppressed. This is referred to as chemical selective water suppression.

The fact that the lipid selective excitation pulse is not selection-selective means that no gradients are applied during its application, so that a large volume is excited. All lipid protons in the homogeneous portion of the field (i.e., the portion of the field that is at 1.5 T) are therefore excited. If a gradient were applied to selectively excite lipid protons in a single section, then water protons in an adjacent section at the low end of the gradient would also be excited. This would interfere with imaging of that section. This technique is, therefore, very sensitive to field inhomogeneities and is effective only for the portions of a sample located near isocenter. However, this technique is simple to perform and does not require any postprocessing of the image data.

There is a more complicated means of obtaining images with the signal from fat or water suppressed. With conventional spin echo sequences, the read gradient is turned on such that the center of the read gradient coincides with the time of the spin echo. Regardless of the difference in precessional frequency between lipid and water protons, the effect of a 180° pulse applied at time TE/2 (after a 90° pulse) is to compensate for all phase differences due to fixed inhomogeneities of the main magnetic field. In an identical manner, the 180° pulse will also compensate for chemical shift differences, which are essentially equivalent to a fixed local field difference.

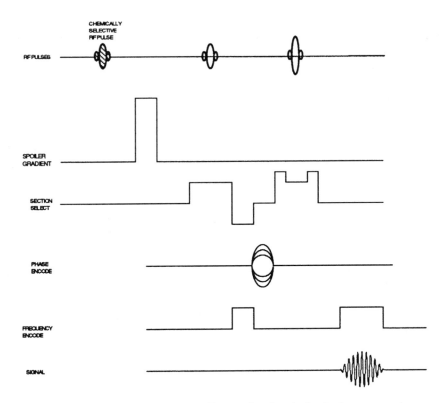

FIGURE 10-24.   Pulse sequence diagram for chemical selective suppression.

Therefore, at time TE after the 180° pulse of a spin echo sequence, fat and water protons will be exactly in phase. Assuming a difference in precessional frequency of 220 Hz between fat and water protons, water protons will precess 220 more cycles than fat protons every second. The time over which water protons precess a half cycle more than fat protons will therefore equal $(1/2)(1/220)$ seconds, which equals 2.3 ms.

Suppose a conventional spin echo imaging sequence is performed, with the spin echo occurring at the center of the frequency-encoding gradient. Then at the center of the signal measurement, lipid and water protons will be in phase. Denote this signal as S_1. Suppose a second imaging sequence is performed, with the center of the frequency-encoding gradient offset by 2.3 ms after the center of the spin echo. Then at the center of this signal measurement, lipid and water protons will be 180° out of phase. Denote this signal as S_2.

If S_1 and S_2 are summed, then the lipid signals will exactly cancel (because they are 180° out of phase) and the remaining signal will represent water only. If S_2 is subtracted from S_1, then the water signal will exactly cancel and the remaining signal will represent lipid only. In this manner, by obtaining two acquisitions, a water-only and a fat-only image can be obtained by addition or subtraction, respectively. Such a technique is usually referred to as the two-point method of **Dixon**. There are several disadvantages to the Dixon method: it requires some image postprocessing, it will only work in the most homogeneous portion of the magnetic field, and it is sensitive to motion between the two acquisitions.

Just like the chemical selective suppression technique described above, the Dixon technique will work only in the most homogeneous portion of the main magnetic field. This can be explained as follows. Suppose the strength of the main field is slightly less than 1.5 T at a particular location. Suppose that water protons are present in this area. These water protons will precess at a frequency less than 63.87 MHz. In fact, suppose the field strength is such that the water protons precess at a frequency of 63.87 MHz − 220 Hz. These water protons will therefore be indistinguishable from lipid protons in the homogeneous portions of the main field, which precess at exactly the same frequency. Both the method of Dixon and the chemical selective suppression techniques will be unable to distinguish such protons.

The two-point method of Dixon can be made less sensitive to field homogeneity by performing additional acquisitions. Suppose the signals S_1 and S_2 are obtained as above. A third acquisition can be acquired with the gradient echo offset by 2.3 ms before the center of the spin echo. Denote this signal by S_3. The signals from the three acquisitions can be used to calculate field inhomogeneities. This can correct for some of the errors described above. This is the three-point Dixon method. However, if severe inhomogeneities are present, even this technique will fail.

To be complete, one final point will be made regarding selective suppression of lipid protons. Lipid protons can be thought of as two distinct chemical species. Lipid protons that are bound to carbon atoms that participate in single bonds with adjacent carbon atoms are referred to as nonolefinic lipid protons. Lipid protons bound to carbon atoms that participate in double or triple bonds are referred to as olefinic lipid protons. Within the human body, the vast majority of lipid protons are non-olefinic. It is the nonolefinic lipid protons that precess at a lower frequency than water protons. The olefinic lipid protons will precess at the same frequency as water protons.

11 Specialized Imaging Sequences

1 GRADIENT ECHO SEQUENCES

Spin echo pulse sequences use a 90° RF excitation pulse followed by a 180° RF pulse at time TE/2 to generate a spin echo at time TE following the original 90° pulse. The purpose of the 90° pulse is to create transverse magnetization (denoted by M_T). The purpose of the 180° pulse is to correct for inhomogeneities in the main magnetic field.

What happens if no 180° pulse is used following the initial 90° pulse? M_T created by the 90° pulse rapidly decays due to T2* relaxation. As described in Chapter 6, the * indicates that decay of M_T results from tissue T2 relaxation as well as dephasing due to inhomogeneities in the main magnetic field and tissue susceptibility differences. The precessing M_T generates a current (the MR signal) in the receiver coil. This signal is usually referred to as the free induction decay, or FID. If nothing else were done, the FID would rapidly (exponentially) diminish in amplitude (Figure 11-1).

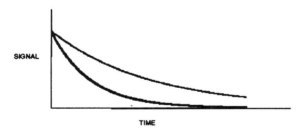

SIGNAL

TIME

FIGURE 11-1. Plot of signal intensity versus time for T2 decay (thin line) and T2* decay (thick line). Note that T2* decay occurs much more rapidly.

The effect of a 180° pulse then is to cause the FID to transiently increase to the value it would have otherwise had if the main magnetic field were perfectly homogeneous and there were no susceptibility differences (Figure 11-2). This transient increase in the FID is referred to as an echo. In order to spatially encode this signal, a phase-encoding gradient is applied prior to the time of the echo and a frequency-encoding gradient is applied during the signal measurement process itself. The timing of the frequency-encoding gradient is such that the peak of the echo occurs at the center of the frequency-encoding gradient. As a result, the echo is symmetric around the center of the frequency-encoding gradient.

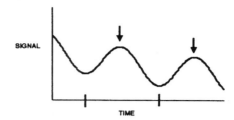

FIGURE 11-2. Plot of signal intensity versus time for a spin echo pulse sequence. The vertical marks along the time axis indicate the time that 180° pulses are applied. The arrows indicate the peak signal intensities (or echoes) following the 180° pulses. The echoes represent the signal that would otherwise have occurred if there were no T2* decay.

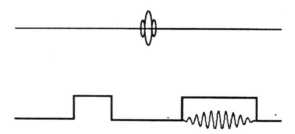

FIGURE 11-3. The read gradient as well as the initial rephasing lobe are of the same polarity because a 180° pulse is applied between the two.

Why is it important that the echo be symmetric around the center of the frequency-encoding gradient? When gradients are first turned on, they are not immediately at full strength and are therefore not perfectly linear. As a result of these imperfections in the earliest portion of a gradient, signal measurements performed at the very beginning of the gradient will have errors. The greater the signal at the beginning of the measurement process, the more significant these errors will be. It is therefore more convenient and more accurate to delay the measurement process such that the maximal signal occurs at the center of the read gradient (and the signal is minimal at the beginning and end of the measurement).

This is accomplished by using a bilobed frequency-encoding gradient, with the signal being measured during the second lobe. The signal is greatly diminished by the first lobe of the gradient, so that at the beginning of the second lobe there is little signal. The signal then grows to a maximum at the center of the second lobe, at which point the dephasing effects of the first lobe have been exactly canceled. The signal again decays during the second half of the second lobe. Because a 180° pulse is applied between the two lobes, the polarity of the two lobes is the same (Figure 11-3).

A second reason for symmetric echo sampling is related to the Fourier transform. The conversion of the voltage as a temporal frequency into a spatial frequency (in k space) prior to Fourier transformation is much easier when the data are sampled using a symmetric echo.

Instead of applying a 180° pulse (following a 90° excitation) and measuring a spin echo, why not measure the FID directly to generate an MR image? In order to measure the FID, the signal must be phase and frequency encoded. The FID can be phase encoded using a gradient identical to the phase-encoding gradient of a spin echo sequence. Suppose a second bilobed gradient (the frequency-encoding gradient) is turned on immediately following (or during) the phase-encoding gradient. The first lobe of this gradient results in dephasing and signal loss. The second lobe is of equal magnitude, twice the duration, and opposite polarity as the first lobe (Figure 11-4). The signal will transiently increase and become maximal (i.e., an echo will form) at the center of the second lobe. Since the echo is generated by a gradient reversal (rather than by a 180° pulse), the above sequence is referred to as a **gradient echo (GRE) sequence**. With the exception that a 180° pulse is not used, gradient echo pulse sequences are nearly identical to spin echo sequences. However, there are important differences.

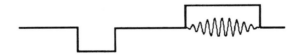

FIGURE 11-4. When using a gradient echo pulse sequence, no 180° pulse is used. Therefore, the read gradient and the rephasing lobe must be of opposite polarity so that the phase changes induced by one are exactly canceled by the other.

Since gradient echo pulse sequences do not use a 180° pulse, decay of M_T following an excitation pulse is dependent on T2* values. It is not possible to obtain true T2-weighted images with most gradient echo pulse sequences. When a relatively long TE is used with a gradient echo pulse sequence, the resulting image contrast is T2* weighted. Therefore, the overall signal generated by gradient echoes is always less than spin echoes (for equal TE and other imaging parameters).

When using a GRE sequence, since no 180° pulse is used, the frequency-encoding gradient can be turned on almost immediately following the excitation pulse. This allows much shorter echo times to be achieved (on the order of 2–3 ms) compared with conventional spin echo sequences. As a result, when short echo times are used, many more sections can be obtained with a GRE sequence compared with a spin echo sequence for a given value of TR.

When using conventional spin echo sequences, the time between excitations (i.e., the TR interval) is usually long enough such that virtually all of the M_T created by one excitation is lost by the time of the next excitation (Figure 11-5). This condition holds provided that TR >> T2. There are several reasons why relatively long TR values are used with conventional spin echo sequences. For T2-weighted images, a long TR is used in order to allow near full recovery of longitudinal magnetization (denoted by M_L) between excitations (Figure 11-6). For T1-weighted images, although a shorter TR is used, the TR must be long enough to allow multiple

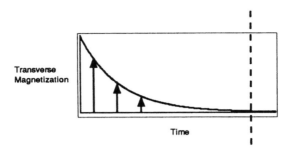

FIGURE 11-5. The arrows represent the amount of persistent transverse magnetization over time following an excitation using a spin echo pulse sequence. This decays in an exponential manner. The dashed vertical line represents the time of the next excitation. There is no persistent transverse magnetization between excitations.

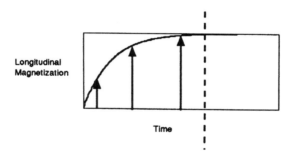

FIGURE 11-6. The arrows represent the amount of longitudinal magnetization over time following an excitation using a spin echo pulse sequence. This grows in an exponential manner. The dashed vertical line represents the time of the next excitation. There is near full recovery of longitudinal magnetization between excitations.

sections to be acquired. Use of the shortest possible TE will maximize the number of sections that can be obtained for a given TR value. However, as discussed above, the minimum TE of spin echo sequences is three to four times that which can be achieved with GRE sequences.

For gradient echo sequences, a much shorter TR is often used (compared with spin echo sequences), so that TR is on the order of T2* or less. Under this condition, there may be significant residual M_T (from prior excitation pulses) at the time of each excitation pulse. GRE sequences that use a long TR are not subject to this effect. Likewise, for conventional spin echo sequences, the TR interval is usually long enough such that there is sufficient time for recovery of M_L between excitation pulses. This condition holds provided that TR is on the order of T1 or greater. However, when using GRE sequences, if TR << T1, there will be very little recovery of M_L between excitations.

To summarize, then, since T2* (or for that matter T2) is almost always much less than T1, the effect of using a TR that is on the order of T2* (which also means that TR << T1) is that there is little recovery of M_L between excitations and there is persistence of M_T between excitations. Consider the effects this has on a gradient echo pulse sequence that uses a short TR.

First, if 90° excitation pulses are used, M_L is entirely converted to M_T. However, at the time of a 90° pulse, the amount of M_L magnetization that is available for conversion into M_T magnetization is dependent upon the recovery of M_L since the prior 90° pulse. When a short TR is used, there is little recovery between excitations (Figure 11-7). Therefore, a relatively weak signal would be produced by such a sequence.

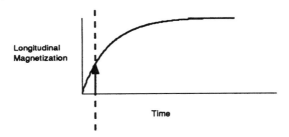

FIGURE 11-7. If the TR interval is short, there is relatively little recovery of longitudinal magnetization between excitations.

Instead of a 90° pulse, suppose a pulse that produces a flip angle of less than 90° were used. This pulse would leave some residual M_L and still create M_T. If the M_L is caused to rotate through an angle of $\alpha°$ with respect to the positive z axis (a so called α pulse, where α is less than 90°), this will create transverse magnetization of magnitude $M_L \sin\alpha$ and leave lognitudinal magnetization of magnitude $M_L \cos\alpha$. For example, $\cos 30° = 0.87$ and $\sin 30° = 0.5$. Therefore, the effect of a 30° pulse is to create transverse magnetization of magnitude $(0.5)M_L$ while leaving longitudinal magnetization of magnitude $(0.87)M_L$ (Figure 11-8). Such a pulse creates significant transverse magnetization while leaving the longitudinal magnetization relatively undisturbed.

In fact, it can be shown mathematically that when using a short TR, maximal echo signal is no longer obtained by using a 90° pulse (as with a spin echo sequence) but instead by using a pulse less than 90°. The angle α is referred to as the **flip angle**. Thus, with short TR gradient echo sequences, a flip angle of less than 90° is often used. Over time, the amount of M_L available (just prior to each excitation pulse) for conversion to M_T will reach an equilibrium state for each voxel. Once equilibrium is established, the same amount of M_T will be created in each voxel following each excitation pulse.

What happens to the residual M_T that does not decay between excitation pulses when using a short TR? Over time, M_T builds up to an equilibrium state (or **steady state**) so that the amount of M_T (in a given voxel) immediately following each excitation pulse becomes constant. It equals the sum of the newly created M_T plus

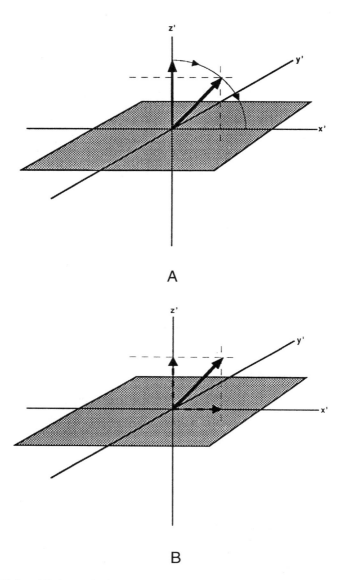

FIGURE 11-8. (A) An excitation pulse causes longitudinal magnetization to be rotated through an angle of 30° with respect to the z′ axis. (B) Following the excitation, residual longitudinal magnetization and newly created transverse magnetization are shown by the dashed arrows along the positive z axis and positive x axis, respectively.

some residual M_T from multiple prior excitations. After each excitation pulse and prior to the signal measurement, M_T in each voxel undergoes T2* decay.

In order for M_T to reach a steady state, a series of 8–12 RF pulses are applied before signal measurements are begun. These are sometimes referred to as discarded data acquisitions and serve to create a steady state of both M_T and M_L.

The B$_1$ field of an excitation pulse causes M$_L$ to rotate into the xy plane. If the RF pulse is at the resonance frequency and is circularly polarized, then the B$_1$ field rotates around the z axis at the resonance frequency. In a frame of reference rotating at the resonance frequency (with coordinates denoted by x', y', and z' to distinguish them from the nonrotating frame of reference), the effect of the B$_1$ field is to cause the net M$_L$ to rotate around the axis of the B$_1$ field.

If, for example, the B$_1$ field is oriented along the positive y' axis in the rotating frame of reference, then M$_L$ will be rotated toward the positive x' axis (Figure 11-9). Therefore, immediately after each excitation pulse, transverse magnetization that is created will be oriented along the positive x' axis. How is this related to the nonrotating (x,y,z) coordinate system? The z' axis is the same as the z axis. The x' and y' axes rotate around the z axis at the resonance frequency.

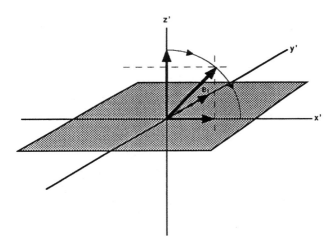

FIGURE 11-9. Longitudinal magnetization is initially oriented along the z' axis. The B$_1$ field is applied along the positive y' axis, which rotates the magnetization toward the x'y' plane. Newly created transverse magnetization will be along the x' axis immediately after the excitation pulse.

As previously noted, the MR system uses a signal at the resonance frequency as a reference. The timing of all excitation pulses, the turning on and off of all gradients, etc., is performed with respect to this reference signal. The position of newly created transverse magnetization immediately following an excitation can also be determined (or specified) with respect to this reference. With proper timing of the excitation pulses, newly created transverse magnetization can have a consistent position (immediately following excitation) from one excitation to the next.

What about the effect of each excitation pulse on residual M$_T$? This is dependent upon the precise orientation of the residual magnetization with respect to the B$_1$ field at the time of excitation. If the B$_1$ field is along the positive y' axis, residual M$_T$ will rotate around this axis. For example, consider residual M$_T$ oriented along the positive x' axis (Figure 11-10). If 90° pulses are used, then the residual M$_T$ will be rotated to the negative z axis (Figure 11-10). In this case, the residual M$_T$ has been completely converted to (negative) longitudinal magnetization. Conversely, if residual M_T is oriented along the negative x' axis (Figure 11-11A), then it will be converted into longitudinal magnetization along the positive z' axis (Figure 11-11B). If the residual M_T is oriented along the y' axis, then the B_1 field will have no effect. For orientations of M_T between the x' and y' axes, the 90° pulse will convert a portion of the residual transverse magnetization into longitudinal magnetization and leave some undisturbed. If an excitation pulse of less than 90° is used, then even residual M_T oriented along the x' axis will not be completely converted into longitudinal magnetization.

What does all this have to do with GRE imaging? For many GRE sequences, TR << T2* and there may be significant residual transverse magnetization in some voxels at the time of each excitation pulse. The timing of the excitation pulses and orientation of the B_1 field with respect to the residual transverse magnetization (of each voxel) can have significant effects on the MR signal. However, the above discussion is pertinent to each individual voxel. Are all voxels the same?

Under ideal conditions (i.e., if the external field were perfectly homogeneous and if there were no differences in magnetic susceptibility between different regions), the signal from all voxels would be exactly in phase except for phase differences induced by the imaging gradients. Therefore, under ideal conditions, if all imaging gradients were exactly balanced at the time of each excitation pulse, residual M_T of all voxels would be exactly in phase at the time of each excitation. A standard GRE pulse sequence using gradients that are balanced at the time of each excitation pulse is shown in Figure 11-12.

Consider what is meant by a balanced gradient. Whenever gradients are on (including the read gradient, the section select gradient, and the phase-encoding gradient), phase changes will be induced along the direction of the gradient. Recall that the section select gradient is bilobed so that the phase changes it induces during excitation are reversed after excitation and before the signal measurement. Likewise, the read gradient is bilobed such that at the center of the read gradient all gradient-induced phase changes are canceled (see Figures 10-18 and 11-4).

When using a spin echo pulse sequence with a relatively long TR, it is necessary to balance gradients only with respect to the signal measurement process. This is because there is no residual transverse magnetization at the time of each excitation. However, when using GRE pulse sequences with a short TR, the effect of imaging gradients on the phase of residual M_T at the time of excitations must also be taken into account. If gradients are not balanced with respect to the time of excitations, then residual M_T in different voxels may not have the same phase at the time of each excitation. The effect of each excitation on the residual M_T of each voxel may then be different.

In order that imaging gradients not induce phase changes in the residual transverse magnetization of each voxel, the gradients must be balanced with respect to each excitation. When using 180° pulses, the conditions are near ideal because the 180° pulses compensate for inhomogeneities in the main field as well as for fixed susceptibility differences. This is not the case with GRE pulse sequences. Even if all of the gradients were balanced with respect to the excitation pulses,

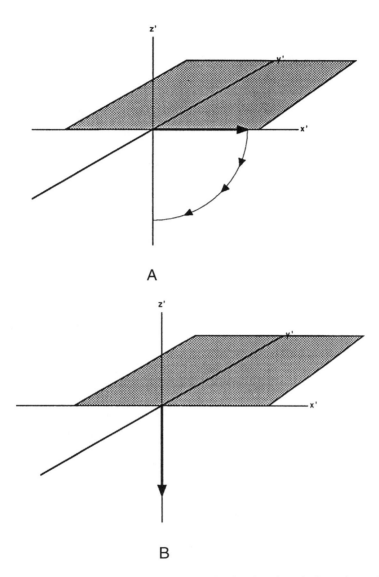

FIGURE 11-10. (A) Residual transverse magnetization is oriented along the positive x′ axis at the time of an excitation pulse. (B) If a 90° pulse is used, then this magnetization will be rotated onto the negative z′ axis.

residual M_T will never be exactly in phase in all of the voxels at the time of each excitation pulse.

On MRI systems, all phase differences are measured with respect to the reference signal at the resonance frequency. Ideally, each excitation pulse is timed so that the transverse magnetization it creates is exactly in phase with the reference signal. The difference in phase between transverse magnetization in a given voxel and the

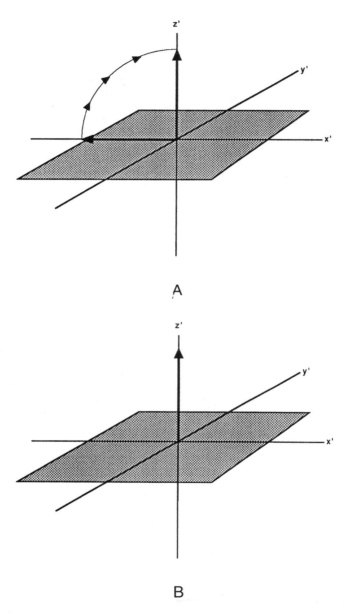

FIGURE 11-11. (A) Residual transverse magnetization is oriented along the negative x′ axis at the time of an excitation pulse. (B) If a 90° pulse is used, then this magnetization will be rotated onto the positive z′ axis.

reference signal is referred to as the phase offset (denoted by the Greek letter psi, ψ). Since the reference signal is at the resonance frequency, the phase offset is sometimes referred to as the **resonance offset**.

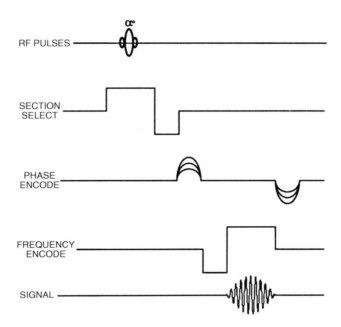

FIGURE 11-12.   Pulse sequence diagram for basic GRE sequence using balanced gradients.

If all gradients were balanced with respect to excitation pulses, then the resonance offset of a given voxel would vary across the FOV depending upon local field inhomogeneities and local susceptibility differences. These resonance offsets would remain constant between excitations. Therefore, some voxels would always have their signal increased by this effect, and others would always have their signal decreased by this effect. This would be manifest as band-like artifact across the reconstructed image.

There are two basic techniques used to prevent these band-like artifacts. The simplest technique is to purposely use gradients that are unbalanced with respect to the timing of the excitation pulses. The read and/or section select gradients are purposely not balanced at the time of each excitation pulse. This introduces phase changes across each voxel such that different portions of the same voxel will have signals with different phases.

If, for example, a voxel were broken into quarters, with the phase of the signal in each quarter offset by $90°$ (note that $90° = 360°/4$), then some portions of each voxel would be in phase with the newly created transverse magnetization and other portions would be out of phase with the newly created transverse magnetization. The strength of the unbalanced gradients can be purposely chosen to cause a $360°$ phase change of the signal across each voxel. The result is that the average resonance offset within each voxel is the same. The strength of the read and section select gradients is not altered between excitations so that this effect also remains constant between different excitations.

The phase-encoding gradient must be rewound between excitations (i.e., it is balanced with respect to excitations) because its magnitude is not constant between excitations. This means that after each signal measurement (and prior to the next signal measurement), a gradient of equal magnitude but opposite polarity to the phase-encoding is applied. This essentially cancels out the phase change induced by each phase-encoding gradient. If not done the effect of the phase-encoding gradient on a given voxel would vary from signal measurement to signal measurement and this would cause image artifact. This image artifact would be caused by an excitation-dependent (i.e., phase-encoding gradient strength-dependent) modulation of the signal amplitude.

The use of unbalanced gradients effectively eliminates the band-like image artifacts that would otherwise occur. It is important to emphasize again that *unbalanced gradients* in the discussion above means unbalanced with respect to the timing of the excitation pulses. The read and section select gradients are always balanced with respect to the signal measurement. Likewise, the phase-encoding gradient is always unbalanced with respect to the signal measurement (in order to provide phase-encoding of the data).

A GRE sequence implemented as described above is usually referred to as a steady-state gradient echo (SSGRE) sequence. This results from the fact that the signal is dependent upon the creation of a steady state of transverse (and longitudinal) magnetization. As described above, the fact that the section select and read gradients are unbalanced at the time of each excitation causes the resonance offset to vary across each voxel. This in essence causes averaging of the resonance offsets across each voxel. This technique is therefore sometimes referred to as ROAST (resonance offset averaging in the steady state). The pulse sequence diagram for a ROAST sequence is shown in Figure 11-13.

SSGRE images can have different types of contrast. GRE images can be relatively T1 weighted, proton density weighted, or T2* weighted. The weighting depends upon the choice of the parameters TR, TE, and flip angle. The type of weighting can be determined by mathematical analysis of the signal intensity equation for GRE imaging. However, it is easy to explain the contrast characteristics of GRE images on a less formal basis as follows:

To minimize T1 weighting, use a small flip angle. A small flip angle causes minimal loss of longitudinal magnetization between excitation pulses. Therefore, regardless of the T1 value (which is the recovery rate of longitudinal magnetization), there is minimal longitudinal magnetization to recover between excitations. All tissues (regardless of their T1 value) will have near full longitudinal magnetization when a small flip angle is used. T1 effects are therefore minimized.

To maximize T1 weighting, use a large flip angle. A large flip angle will cause significant loss of longitudinal magnetization between excitation pulses. Therefore, the degree of recovery of longitudinal magnetization between excitation pulses will depend upon the T1 of each tissue. Hence the signal of each tissue will depend upon its T1 value.

To minimize T2* weighting, use a short TE. A short TE will minimize loss of transverse magnetization prior to signal measurement. That is, by using a short TE, no tissues will undergo significant loss of transverse magnetization prior to mea-

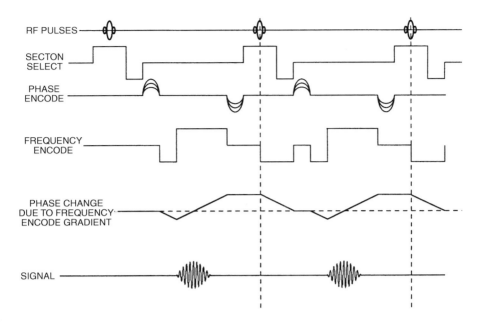

FIGURE 11-13. Pulse sequence diagram for SSGRE sequence. The frequency encoding gradient is purposely unbalanced at the time of the excitation pulses. Phase changes induced by the frequency-encoding gradient are shown at the bottom of the diagram.

surement regardless of their T2*. To maximize T2* weighting, use a long TE. A long TE will allow differential signal loss between tissues depending on their T2* value.

The effect of TR is more complex. If TR is on the order of T2* or less for most tissues being imaged, then many voxels will have significant residual transverse magnetization between excitation pulses. For this range of TR values, a relatively longer TR will enhance T2* weighting. If, however, the TR is long enough, most tissues will lose almost all transverse magnetization between excitation pulses. Under this circumstance, TR >> T2* and small changes in TR will not have significant effects because there will be near complete loss of transverse magnetization between excitation pulses anyway.

Thus, for SSGRE imaging we have the following general guidelines:

1. To generate T1 weighting, use a large flip angle, a short TE, and a long TR (i.e., a TR >> T2*).
2. To generate T2* weighting, use a small flip angle, a long TE, and a short TR (i.e., a TR on the order of T2* or less).
3. To generate proton density weighting, use a small flip angle, a short TE, and a long TR.

There is a second method of dealing with the residual transverse magnetization when using GRE sequences. After each signal measurement, strong gradients can be purposely applied to dephase persistent transverse magnetization. These gradients prevent the establishment of a steady state. Under such conditions, the signal emitted from each voxel following an excitation will reflect only the transverse magnetization created by that excitation. This can effectively remove T2* weighting from the image (provided that a short TE is used). Since the dephasing gradients are usually referred to as spoiler gradients, this technique is referred to as a **spoiled GRE** sequence.

In reality, most spoiled GRE sequences use RF spoiling instead of gradient spoiling. For SSGRE sequences, the excitation pulses are timed such that the transverse magnetization created following each excitation pulse maintains a constant phase relationship with the reference signal. If instead of always keeping this phase the same, the excitation pulses are timed such that the phase is random, then a significant steady-state transverse magnetization will not build up. This is referred to as **RF spoiling**, because it is the random phase of the RF excitation pulses that act to spoil the phase coherence of the residual transverse magnetization.

Spoiled GRE sequences usually use a short TE and a large flip angle to provide images with contrast similar to conventional spin echo T1-weighted images. Because these sequences do not allow a steady state to develop, spoiled GRE sequences cannot develop true T2*-weighted contrast.

Some of the contrast characteristics of GRE sequences are unique. GRE images are sensitive to magnetic susceptibility differences. That is, near interfaces of tissues with different magnetic susceptibility, there will be significant signal loss or a near signal void. This is why hemosiderin has a dark appearance on GRE images (due to its iron content, hemosiderin has a much greater magnetic susceptibility than other tissues, which causes a stronger local field). Likewise, in bone marrow there are local field differences due to marrow adjacent to cortical bone. Cortical bone contains little water and has a different susceptibility than the marrow. As a result, marrow shows relatively low signal on GRE sequences.

Another unique characteristic of GRE images is the appearance of lipid/water interfaces. When exposed to the same external magnetic field strength, lipid protons precess slightly slower than water protons. At 1.5 T, water protons precess at a rate 220 Hz faster than lipid protons. This corresponds to water protons precessing one half cycle more than lipid protons every 2.3 ms.

If a voxel contains both water and lipid protons, the signals from the water and lipid protons will be out of phase 2.3 ms following an excitation pulse, in phase 4.6 ms following an excitation pulse, out of phase 6.9 ms following an excitation pulse, and so on. If the TE of a GRE sequence happens to be at or near an even multiple of 2.3 ms, then the signal from voxels that contain both water and lipid protons will be unaffected (Figure 11-14). However, if the TE of a GRE sequence happens to be at or near 2.3 ms or any odd multiple of 2.3 ms , then the signal from voxels that contain both water and lipid protons will be greatly diminished. This is manifest as a dark line at lipid/water interfaces on GRE sequences when TE is near one of the above values (Figure 11-15). This effect is not seen with spin echo pulse sequences because the 180° pulse compensates for the difference in precessional frequency between water and lipid protons.

A question that naturally arises is, can the spin echo technique be used with a very short TR and a flip angle of less than 90°? The answer is yes. However, the

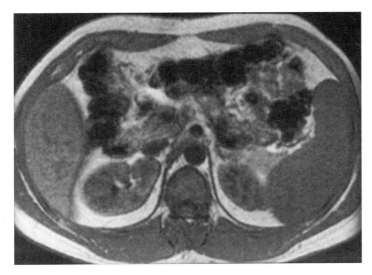

FIGURE 11-14. GRE image obtained with an echo time of 4.5 ms (fat and water protons in phase) through the lower abdomen. There is no etching around the margins of the liver or spleen.

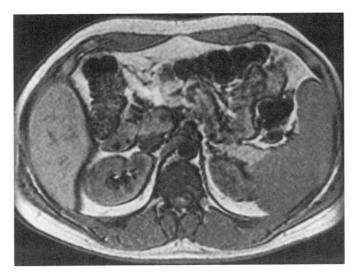

FIGURE 11-15. GRE image obtained at same level as in Figure 11-14 but with an echo time of 2.3 ms (fat and water protons out of phase). The margins of the liver, spleen, kidneys, and anterior abdominal muscles are dark, giving a so called etched appearance.

strategy is slightly different than that used for GRE sequences. Suppose an excitation pulse ($0 < \alpha < 90°$) is followed by a 180° pulse. The residual longitudinal magnetization following the α pulse will be oriented along the positive z′ axis (i.e., along

the external field direction) (Figure 11-16). Following the 180° pulse, this magnetization will be rotated to the negative z' axis. The longitudinal magnetization would
then recover toward the positive z axis.

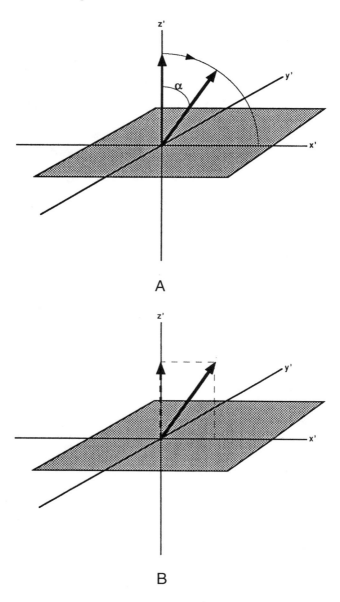

FIGURE 11-16. (A) Prior to an excitation pulse, net magnetization is along the positive z
axis. An α° RF pulse (with α° < 90°) rotates the net longitudinal magnetization toward the
positive x' axis. (B) Following the excitation pulse, the net longitudinal magnetization has
been reduced (shown by the dashed arrow) but is still oriented along the positive z axis.

It would be more efficient to use an excitation pulse of $(180 - \alpha)°$. This will create the same degree of transverse magnetization as an α pulse, but will create longitudinal magnetization oriented along the negative z′ axis (Figure 11-17). Following a 180° pulse this longitudinal magnetization will be rotated to the positive z′ axis. The net longitudinal magnetization will then increase until the time of the next $(180° - \alpha)$ pulse.

Such a sequence could certainly be used to generate spin echo images with a very short TR. A small value of α and a long TE could be used to generate T2-weighted images. The minimum TR of such a sequence would be on the order of 60–100 ms because it must exceed the TE. In addition, only one section could be acquired during such a TR interval and the S/N of these images would be poor. T1-weighted images could be acquired by using a large flip angle and a short TE. The minimum TR of such a sequence would exceed that of a similar GRE sequence because it takes more time to use a 180° pulse to generate an echo.

1.1 STIMULATED ECHOES

As noted above, when imaging with GRE sequences, if TR < T2*, transverse magnetization persists between excitation pulses. This leads to an additional phenomenon when sequential excitation pulses of less than 180° are used. Echoes are created that differ from those created by gradients applied to the FID. These are actually a form of spin echo and are referred to as stimulated echoes. How do these stimulated echoes arise?

Suppose a collection of protons is placed in an external magnetic field (B_0). If, for example, a 90° excitation pulse is applied, M_T is created within each voxel. The precessional frequency of M_T is proportional to the local field strength. If the field were perfectly homogeneous, then the local field strength at all locations would be B_0. However, due to field inhomogeneities, at some points the field strength will be greater or less than B_0.

If the local field strength equals B_0, the precessional frequency of M_T will equal ω_0. If the local field strength is less than B_0, the precessional frequency of M_T will equal $\omega_0 - \Delta\omega$ (for some value $\Delta\omega$), and, similarly, if the local field strength is greater than B_0, the precessional frequency of M_T will equal $\omega_0 + \Delta\omega$ (for some value $\Delta\omega$).

The effect of the B_1 field of an RF excitation pulse is to rotate the net magnetization. The axis of rotation is dependent upon the orientation of B_1. If the B_1 field is oriented along the positive y′ axis and a 90° pulse is applied, M_L will be completely converted into M_T and the newly created M_T will be oriented along the positive x′ axis (Figure 11-18A and B). While the axis of rotation itself is not important, each excitation pulse is timed such that it rotates the magnetization within a sample around the same axis each time. In the following discussion, it will be assumed that for each excitation, the B_1 field is along the positive y′ axis.

Consider the effect of sequential 90° excitation pulses on a pair of voxels whose transverse magnetization has precessional frequencies $\omega_0 + \Delta\omega$ and $\omega_0 - \omega$. The entire sample can be thought of as consisting of such pairs of voxels with each pair having a different value of $\Delta\omega$. Denote the transverse magnetization in the voxel with precessional frequency $\omega_0 + \Delta\omega$ as M_{TF} (the _f_aster voxel) and the transverse

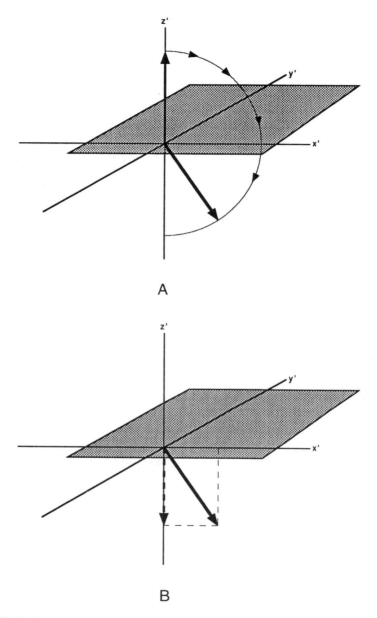

FIGURE 11-17. (A) Prior to an excitation pulse, net magnetization is along the positive z axis. An $(180 - \alpha)°$ RF pulse (with $\alpha° < 90°$) rotates the net longitudinal magnetization past the positive x′ axis. (B) Following the excitation pulse, the net longitudinal magnetization (shown by the dashed arrow) is now oriented along the negative z axis.

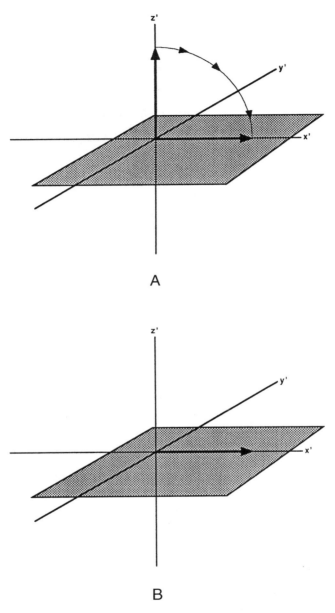

A

B

FIGURE 11-18. (A) A 90° excitation pulse is applied, which rotates the longitudinal magnetization onto the x′ axis. (B) Immediately following the excitation pulse, transverse magnetization is oriented along the positive x′ axis.

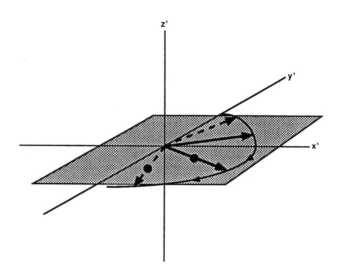

FIGURE 11-19. Over time, the transverse magnetization in each pair of voxels will get out of phase. The solid arrows represent two voxels with a small phase difference between their transverse magnetization and the dashed arrows represent two voxels with a large phase difference between their transverse magnetization. The faster transverse magnetization of each pair is shown with a solid circle. In the (x,y,z) coordinate system, these vectors (representing transverse magnetization) rotate clockwise around the z axis (as shown by the small arrowheads).

magnetization in the voxel with precessional frequency $\omega_0 - \omega$ as M_{TS} (the slower voxel).

Let the first 90° RF pulse be applied at time t = 0. Immediately following this pulse, all of the longitudinal magnetization will be converted to transverse magnetization and the transverse magnetization within each voxel will be oriented along the positive x′ axis. M_{TF} will precess at frequency $\omega_0 + \Delta\omega$ and M_{TS} will precess at frequency $\omega_0 - \omega$. These will begin to get out of phase. As they get out of phase, the net signal emitted by the pair will diminish over time. Suppose that at time T, these two voxels are $\Delta\phi$ out of phase, with M_{TF} having acquired a relative positive phase with respect to M_{TS} (Figure 11-19). Consider the following two scenarios:

1. A 180° pulse is applied at time T. This will rotate all transverse magnetization 180° around the y′ axis. This changes the phase relationship of the voxels such that M_{TF} now has a negative phase $(-\Delta\phi)$ with respect to M_{TS} (Figure 11-20). The precessional frequency of each voxel remains unchanged. Therefore, after another interval of time T has elapsed (i.e., at time t = 2T), M_{TF} will acquire an additional positive phase $+\Delta\phi$ with respect to M_{TF}. The total phase difference between M_{TF} and M_{TS} at time t = 2T is therefore $(-\Delta\phi) + (+\Delta\phi) = 0$. At time t = 2T, the transverse magnetization in the two voxels will once again be in phase and their

signal will be maximal. The effect is the same for all such pairs of voxels regardless of the value of $\Delta\phi$. This is what occurs with a conventional spin echo sequence.

2. A 90° pulse is applied at time t = T. This will rotate all transverse magnetization 90° around the y' axis (Figure 11-21A). This will convert some transverse magnetization into longitudinal magnetization. The degree of conversion will depend upon the orientation of the transverse magnetization with respect to the axis of rotation (the y' axis) at the time of the excitation pulse. If the transverse magnetization is oriented along the x' axis at the time of the excitation pulse, it will be completely converted into longitudinal magnetization. If the transverse magnetization is oriented along the y' axis at the time of the excitation pulse it will be unaffected.

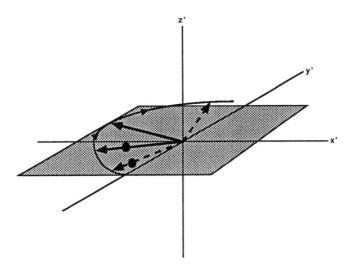

FIGURE 11-20. A 180° RF pulse is applied (at the time shown in Figure 11-19) that rotates all transverse magnetization 180° around the y' axis. This inverts the relationship of each pair of transverse magnetization. The faster transverse magnetization of each pair (indicated by the solid circle) is now "behind" the slower transverse magnetization. All transverse magnetization continues to rotate clockwise around the z' axis as shown by the small arrowheads. This is what happens with a standard spin echo pulse sequence when a 90° pulse is followed by a 180° pulse.

For argument's sake, assume that at time t = T, $\Delta\phi$, the phase difference between M_{TF} and M_{TS}, is between 0° and 180°, as in Figure 11-19. Furthermore, suppose that at the time of the second 90° pulse M_{TS} is oriented at angle $(180° - \Delta\phi)/2$ with respect to the positive y' axis, and that M_{TF} is oriented at an angle $(180° - \Delta\phi/2)$ with respect to the negative y' axis. Both are within the x'y' plane at the time of the pulse. The second 90° pulse will partially rotate both net magnetizations out of the transverse plane. Immediately following the second 90° pulse, each will have a

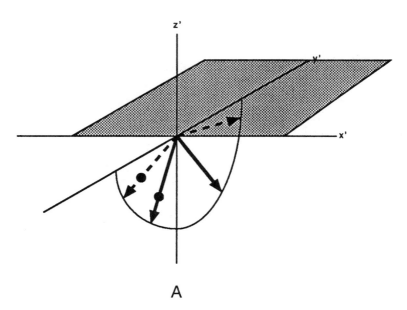

A

FIGURE 11-21A. Instead of applying a 180° pulse at time t = T, as in Figure 11-20, a 90° RF pulse is applied which rotates all transverse magnetization 90° around the y′ axis. Immediately after this 90° pulse, all magnetization will be within the y′z′ plane as shown.

component of transverse magnetization and longitudinal magnetization (Figures 11-21B, C, D, and E).

The transverse component of M_{TF} will be oriented along the negative y′ axis, and the transverse component of M_{TS} will be oriented along the positive y′ axis. Since these components are of equal magnitude but opposite direction, the net transverse magnetization will be zero immediately after the second 90° pulse (Figures 11-21D and E). This is true for all pairs of voxels regardless of Δφ. However, some of the transverse magnetization will be converted into longitudinal magnetization (Figure 11-21F). When additional 90° excitation pulses are applied, this longitudinal magnetization can be reconverted into transverse magnetization. It is therefore sometimes referred to as **stored** longitudinal magnetization.

Therefore, the effect of the second 90° pulse is to cause the transverse components of magnetization of each pair of voxels to be 180° out of phase (immediately following the pulse). At time t = 2T, the phase difference of the transverse components will be 180° − Δφ (Figure 11-21G). Unlike the situation of a 90° pulse followed by a 180° pulse, the phase difference at time t = 2T is dependent on Δφ. In fact, the greater the phase change between a pair of voxels at the time of the second 90° pulse, the smaller the phase change at time t = 2T. That is, those voxels most out of phase at the time of the second 90° pulse will be most in phase at time t = 2T.

This partial to complete rephasing of the transverse components of each pair of voxels at time t = 2T will give rise to an echo. Since the transverse components in different pairs of voxels are not all exactly in phase, the magnitude of the echo at t

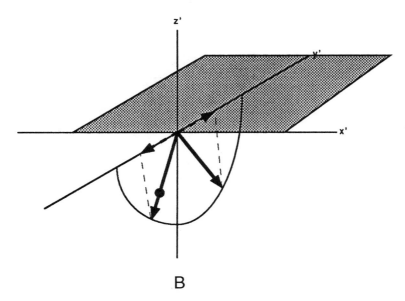

B

FIGURE 11-21B. The components of transverse magnetization of the first pair of vectors are shown by the dashed arrows which are oriented along the positive and negative y′ axis. These components are of equal magnitude but opposite direction. The net transverse magnetization of the first pair immediately following the second 90° pulse is therefore zero.

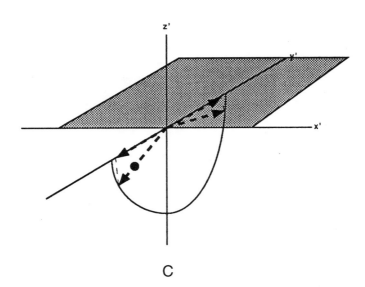

C

FIGURE 11-21C. The components of transverse magnetization of the second pair of vectors are shown by the dashed arrows which are oriented along the positive and negative y′ axis. These components are of equal magnitude but opposite direction. The net transverse magnetization of the second pair immediately following the second 90° pulse is therefore also equal to zero.

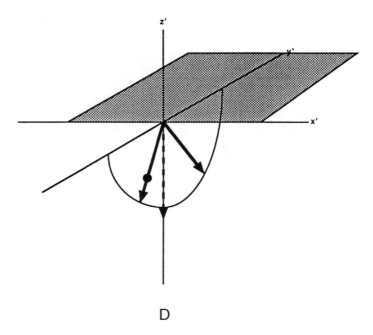

D

FIGURE 11-21D.   The components of longitudinal magnetization of the first pair of vectors are both oriented along the negative z axis. The net longitudinal magnetization of this pair of vectors is shown by the dashed arrow along the negative z′ axis.

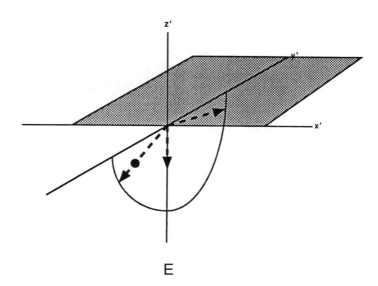

E

FIGURE 11-21E.   The components of longitudinal magnetization of the second pair of vectors are oriented along the negative z axis. The net longitudinal magnetization of this pair of is shown by the dashed arrow along the negative z′ axis.

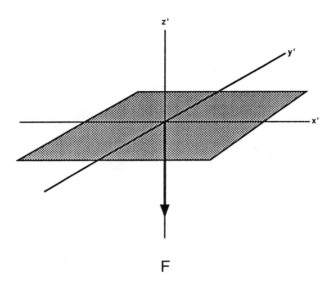

F

FIGURE 11-21F. For each pair of vectors, the net transverse magnetization is zero. Likewise, for each pair of vectors, the net longitudinal magnetization points along the negative z′ axis. This figure shows the overall net magnetization from all such pairs immediately following the second 90° pulse.

= 2T caused by two 90° pulses is less than that caused by a 90° pulse followed by a 180° pulse. Such an echo, however, is still referred to as a spin echo.

In a similar manner, if additional 90° pulses are applied, additional echoes will be generated. The additional echoes (beyond the first echo) are referred to as **stimulated echoes**. These echoes can be thought of as being formed by converting the stored longitudinal magnetization (from prior 90° pulses) back into transverse magnetization. The stimulated echo signal will be maximal at times 3T, 4T, etc. Since T is the time between excitation pulses, T = TR. Therefore, the stimulated echoes will be centered around the time of the excitation pulses.

In fact, if multiple α pulses (rather than 90° pulses) are applied consecutively with $0 < \alpha < 180°$, many stimulated echoes will be generated. Therefore, whenever multiple RF pulses of less than 180° are applied to a sample, stimulated echoes will be generated. The time of occurrence of the stimulated echoes will be centered around the time of application of the excitation pulses.

To review, then, whenever multiple RF pulses are used such that residual transverse magnetization persists between excitations, both an FID signal and stimulated echoes will result. The FID is maximal immediately following each excitation pulse. The stimulated echo is maximal at the time just before each excitation pulse. Residual transverse magnetization will persist between excitation pulses unless TR >> T2*. For most GRE sequences with a short TR, TR is not significantly greater than T2* and stimulated echoes will occur.

What happens when both a gradient echo and a stimulated echo occur? The gradient echo is centered around the read gradient. The stimulated echo is centered

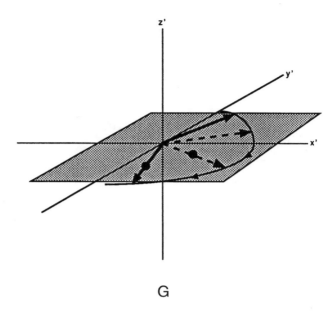

G

FIGURE 11-21G. At time t = 2T, the components of transverse magnetization have changed their orientations as shown. Note that the pair of vectors (solid arrows) that had the smaller phase difference immediately following the second 90° pulse now have the larger phase difference. On the other hand, the pair of vectors (dashed arrows) that had the larger phase difference immediately following the second 90° pulse now have the smaller phase difference. Unlike a standard spin echo pulse sequence where the 180° pulse causes all pairs of transverse magnetization to be exactly in phase at the time of an echo, each pair of transverse magnetization is only partially in phase at the time of the echo. The degree to which each pair is in phase is inversely related to the phase difference at the time of the second 90° pulse.

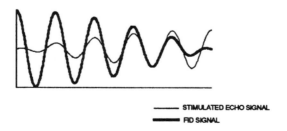

——— STIMULATED ECHO SIGNAL
■■■■■ FID SIGNAL

FIGURE 11-22. As the FID signal decays (thick solid graph), the stimulated echo signal (thin solid graph) increases in amplitude.

around the excitation pulses (Figure 11-22). In most circumstances, the two echoes do not overlap and can be measured separately. Ordinarily, only the gradient echo is measured. This is because the timing of the stimulated echo coincides with the excitation pulses and it is therefore not convenient to measure the stimulated echo.

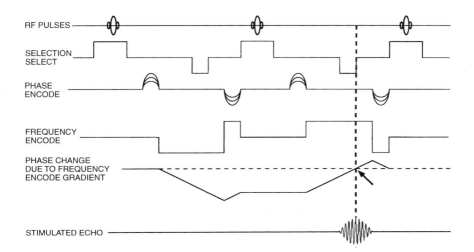

FIGURE 11-23.   The phase changes due to the frequency-encoding gradient only are shown. Note that these phase changes become zero just prior to the third excitation pulse (shown by the arrow and the dashed line). The stimulated echo will be maximal at this point.

However, a gradient echo pulse sequence can be performed so that the stimulated echoes can be measured instead of the FID. The key to understanding this is to examine the effect of the section selective and read gradients on the gradient echo and the stimulated echo.

The gradient echo of a SSGRE sequence is formed by using a balanced section select gradient (balanced with respect to the timing of the excitation pulse) followed by a bilobed read gradient. The read gradient is balanced halfway through the second lobe. This balancing of the read gradient occurs early in the interval between successive excitation pulses. Since the FID quickly decays (and is maximum immediately following an excitation), the earlier the gradient echo is formed (and read) after an excitation, the greater its signal will be. On the other hand, a stimulated echo will have its peak immediately before an excitation. Hence, the strength of the stimulated echo will usually be negligible (but present) at the time that a gradient echo is typically measured.

How can the stimulated echo be measured instead of the FID echo? Consider three 90° excitation pulses applied at times t = 0, t = TR, and t = 2TR. Change the section select gradients so that the rephasing lobe occurs just prior to (rather than just after) each excitation pulse (Figure 11-23). Then over the interval from t = 0 to t = TR (and from t = TR to t = 2TR) the section select gradient from one excitation pulse will not be balanced until just prior to the next excitation. Next, change the read gradient such that the first lobe is considerably longer than the second lobe. Then over the interval from t = 0 to t = TR, this gradient will not be balanced. As a result, the echo from the FID will be greatly diminished.

If we then reverse the direction of the lobes of the read gradient for the interval from t = TR to t = 2TR, then this gradient will be balanced just prior to the third excitation (Figure 11-23). The time at which this occurs can be adjusted by the timing of turning on the read gradient. Denote this interval of time by Δt. Since the stimulated echo peaks at this time, if we center the signal measurement at TR $-\Delta t$, we will be measuring the stimulated echo. It is important to note that the FID echo signal is still present, but it peaks just after each excitation pulse and then rapidly falls off.

Since the gradients are balanced at time Δt prior to the third excitation, the effective echo time for the stimulated echo will be 2TR $-\Delta t$. As noted above, Δt is controlled by the timing of the read gradient. Such a sequence is usually referred to as steadystate free precession (SSFP). The advantage of measuring the stimulated echo is that it is a form of spin echo (not a GRE) and therefore can provide images with T2 contrast rather than T2* contrast. This is achieved by using a small flip angle to reduce T1 weighting.

Although it seems that a stimulated echo will form only just before every third excitation, once the first three excitations have been applied, stimulated echoes will actually form prior to each excitation. For example, the first stimulated echo will occur just prior to excitation 3 as a result of excitations 1 and 2. The second stimulated echo will occur just prior to excitation 4 as a result of excitations 2 and 3. The third stimulated echo will occur just prior to excitation 5 as a result of excitations 3 and 4, and so on. Prior to an actual imaging sequence, multiple excitation pulses are applied without performing signal measurement in order to allow the system to achieve a steady state.

With the implementation of the SSFP sequence as described above, the gradient echo is actually offset from the spin echo by time Δt in order that it be more convenient to measure. Therefore, the SSFP sequence will actually have a small degree of T2* weighting, proportional to $e^{-\Delta t/T2*}$. Since Δt is very small, the amount of T2* weighting is minimal.

By a more clever arrangement of the gradients, a sequence that measures both the gradient echo and the stimulated echo can be designed.

Although not readily apparent, stimulated echoes can also arise when a sample is exposed to multiple closely spaced consecutive 180° pulses. This results from the fact that when a section of tissue is exposed to a 180° pulse, the edges of the section actually experience less than a 180° pulse. Due to imperfections in the pulses, only the center of the section actually experiences a true 180° pulse. This is because pulse profiles are never perfectly rectangular.

This has important implications when performing fast spin echo pulse sequences. As a series of 180° pulses is applied, many stimulated echoes will be generated. The signal from the stimulated echoes will peak at the time of the 180° pulses. However, there will be some signal from these stimulated echoes at the time of signal measurement. The closer the spacing of the 180° pulses, the greater will be the contribution from the stimulated echoes.

In fast spin echo sequences, as with SSGRE sequences, phase rewinder gradients are used between excitations. This results in all of the stimulated echoes being in phase with each other and with the spin echo signal. In fact, when the spacing between 180° pulses of a fast spin echo sequence is made as short as possible, the contribution to the overall signal from stimulated echoes will be substantial.

1.2 Volume Imaging

When using conventional spin echo or GRE sequences, the minimum section thickness that can be achieved has a lower limit. In part, this is due to the fact that the section select gradient strength is inversely proportional to the section thickness. This means that to acquire thinner sections, the section select gradient strength has to be increased. Therefore, the minimum section thickness depends on the maximum section select gradient strength that the gradient amplifiers can produce.

The bandwidth of section selective excitation pulses is usually fixed. Suppose this bandwidth is ΔBW_S. When a section of tissue is selectively excited, the strength of the section select gradient is adjusted so that the difference in precessional frequency of protons from one side of the section to the other is equal to ΔBW_S. Alternatively, thinner sections could be obtained by use of an excitation pulse with a smaller value of ΔBW_S. However, there is a penalty for this.

With most conventional spin echo sequences, when a section of tissue is excited (in the presence of the section select gradient), the center frequency of the excitation pulse is chosen to coincide with the precessional frequency of water protons at the center of the section. At 1.5 T, lipid protons will precess at a frequency 220 Hz less than water protons. As a result, the actual region of lipid excited will be shifted along the section select direction causing a misexcitation of the lipid protons.

Therefore, lipid within a small portion of the section to be excited on the low-frequency side of the section select gradient will remain unexcited. Similarly, lipid present within a small portion beyond the section to be excited on the high-frequency side of the section select gradient will be excited and contribute to the received signal. The greater this misexcitation, the more the image will be distorted.

The thickness of the portion of lipid within a section that remains unexcited (which equals the thickness of the portion of lipid outside of a section that is excited) expressed as a fraction of section thickness is equal to $(220/\Delta BW_S)$. The lower the value of ΔBW_S, the greater this fraction. Therefore, the lower the value of ΔBW_S, the greater the resulting image distortion. This factor places a lower limit on the value of ΔBW_S that can practically be used. Most imaging systems use the minimum value of ΔB_S that results in an acceptable level of distortion from this misexcitation effect. This will be discussed in greater detail in the chapter on imaging artifacts (Chapter 14).

The S/N of an image is directly proportional to the section thickness. Therefore, as thinner sections are used, the S/N will be diminished. In order to maintain the S/N at acceptable levels when very thin sections are used (without sacrificing in-plane resolution), the NSA would have to be substantially increased.

For example, suppose conventional spin echo images were obtained with the following parameters: section thickness = 5 mm, square FOV = L, N_f = number of frequency encodings, and N_p = number of phase-encodings. Then the S/N is proportional to $[(5L^2) \times (\sqrt{NSA})]/[(\sqrt{N_p}) \times N_f]$. If in-plane resolution is maintained constant (i.e., L, N_p, and N_f are fixed) and the section thickness is decreased to 1 mm, then the S/N would be diminished by a factor of 5. The only way to compensate for this while keeping the S/N constant is to increase the NSA by a factor of 25. This would result in an increase of imaging time by a factor of 25. Although the

TR could be reduced to diminish imaging time, it can be reduced only by a small amount since the range of TR values for conventional spin echo T1- and T2-weighted images is limited.

Therefore, the minimum section thickness that can be achieved using conventional spin echo pulse sequences is limited by the maximum section select gradient strength and S/N considerations. When multiplanar imaging is performed using spin echo or gradient echo pulse sequences, multiple sections are excited in sequential manner during each TR interval. The volume of tissue imaged consists of a stack of sections with a small intersection gap. A section select gradient is used to selectively excite one section at a time. The selective excitation allows the signal from different sections to be distinguished.

Suppose the section select gradient is decreased in strength so that a single excitation pulse excites the entire volume of tissue to be imaged. The signal can still be encoded in the plane of section by using standard phase and frequency encoding. A new means of spatially encoding the signal along the section select direction (other than exciting one section at a time, measuring the signal, and then exciting the next section) is needed. The simplest means of accomplishing this is to apply an additional phase-encoding gradient along the section select direction. The number of distinct phase-encoding gradients required along the section select direction is equal to the number of desired sections. Denote the number of phase-encoding gradients along the section select direction as N_s.

In order to generate an image from a volume acquisition, we must now perform a three-dimensional Fourier transform. k space now has three axes: k_x, k_y, and k_z. The signal must be sampled along all three axes. The number of samples along k_x is equal to N_f, the number of samples along k_y is equal to N_p, and the number of samples along k_z is equal to N_s. Since each sample along a given axis must be obtained with the values along the other axes held constant, the total number of samples required for a volume acquisition is equal to $N_f \times N_p \times N_s$. That is, N_f frequency samples are obtained during each signal measurement for each pair of values of the in-plane and section select phase-encoding gradient strengths.

For example, with a multisection conventional spin echo acquisition (i.e., a two-dimensional acquisition), if $N_p = 128$ and NSA $= 1$, then 128 signal measurements are performed, each with a different strength of the phase-encoding gradient. On the other hand, suppose a volume acquisition is performed with $N_p = 128$, $N_s = 2$, and NSA $= 1$. For each of the two values of the section select phase-encoding gradient strength, 128 signal measurements must be performed, each with a different value of the in-plane phase-encoding gradient strength. That is, 256 signal measurements must be performed.

Therefore, the total imaging time for a volume acquisition is equal to TR $\times$ NSA $\times N_p \times N_s$. If the volume of tissue excited is of length V along the section select direction, then the section thickness (T) is equal to V/N_s. Compared with a two-dimensional acquisition, the total number of excitations performed is multiplied by the factor N_s. This multiplies the S/N by a factor of $\sqrt{N_s}$. The SNR of a volume acquisition is proportional to $[(L_f \times L_p) \times T \times \sqrt{NSA} \times \sqrt{N_s}]/(N_f \times \sqrt{N_p})$, all other factors affecting S/N held constant. Therefore, for equal in-plane resolution, NSA, and section thickness, a volume acquisition will have SNR improved by a factor of

$\sqrt{N_s}$ compared with a two-dimensional acquisition. Hence, volume acquisitions are an effective means of obtaining very thin sections with good S/N.

When an individual section of tissue is imaged, if any tissue is present outside of the FOV along the phase-encoding direction, phase wraparound artifact would occur. This can be reduced by using an imaging option that doubles the FOV along the phase-encoding direction. At the same time, the NSA is reduced by half in order to maintain imaging time constant (see Chapter 10).

When a volume acquisition is performed, there will be excitation of a small amount of tissue on either side of the volume along the section select direction. Since the signal along the section select direction is phase encoded, the signal emitted by this tissue (outside of the volume of interest) may be wrapped into the ends of the volume. Hence, the end sections of a volume acquisition would suffer from wraparound artifact. In order to prevent wraparound artifact in the end sections of a volume acquisition, several sections at each end of the volume are usually discarded. This is equivalent to performing extra phase-encoding steps along the section select direction of a volume acquisition.

As noted above, for conventional spin echo sequences and GRE sequences, the imaging time of a volume acquisition is given by $TR \times NSA \times N_p \times N_s$. Therefore, volume acquisitions are usually performed only with GRE sequences with as short a TR as possible. With fast spin echo sequences (described below), the imaging time of a volume acquisition is given by $TR \times NSA \times N_p \times N_s/ETL$, where ETL is the echo train length. This assumes that fast spin echo phase-encoding is performed along one direction only. With such an approach, volume imaging can be performed in reasonable periods of time using spin echoes.

2   INVERSION RECOVERY SEQUENCES

An inversion recovery sequence is identical to a conventional spin echo sequence with the exception of the addition of a 180° pulse prior to the 90° pulse. The effect of the first 180° pulse (referred to as an inversion pulse) is to invert the longitudinal magnetization aligned with the B_0 field so that it becomes aligned against the B_0 field. The longitudinal magnetization is then allowed to recover until the time of the 90° pulse. The degree of recovery in each voxel is dependent upon the T1 of the tissue contained in that voxel. The time between the 180° and the 90° pulse is referred to as **TI** (time of inversion) or **tau** (since it is sometimes denoted by the Greek letter τ) The inversion recovery sequence therefore uses a 180° pulse, followed after a time TI by a 90° pulse, followed after another time TE/2 by a 180° pulse (Figure 11-24A).

Tissues with a short T1 will recover their longitudinal magnetization relatively quickly. Tissues with a long T1 recover their longitudinal magnetization relatively slowly. By choosing TI such that a tissue has zero net longitudinal magnetization at the time of the 90° pulse, no transverse magnetization will be created and therefore this tissue will produce no signal (Figure 11-24B).

Inversion recovery sequences that use a relatively short TI are referred to as STIR (which stands for short TI inversion recovery) sequences. These sequences are useful because by appropriate choice of TI, the signal from fat can be suppressed.

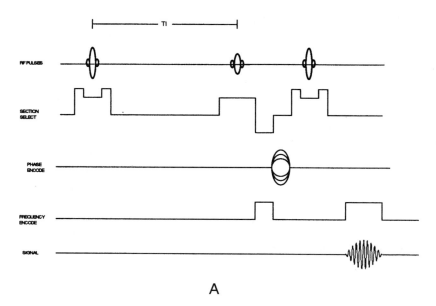

A

FIGURE 11-24A. The short TI inversion recovery (STIR) pulse diagram is the same as that for a conventional spin echo pulse sequence except for the addition of a 180° pulse prior to the 90° pulse.

It is important to note that signal from any tissue with the same T1 as fat (e.g., certain stages of evolving hematoma) will also be suppressed. Therefore, STIR sequences cannot be used to distinguish fat from blood or other proteinaceous fluid that may have a T1 comparable to fat.

Most pathologic abnormalities have a long T1 relaxation time and a long T2 relaxation time. Thus, on conventional spin echo sequences, most pathologic lesions appear relatively hypointense on T1-weighted images and relatively hyperintense on T2-weighted images. The increased signal on T2-weighted sequences is due solely to increased T2.

On STIR sequences, the long T1 of most pathologic abnormalities will result in increased signal. By also choosing a long TE, the long T2 of most pathologic abnormalities will result in increased signal. Thus, by using an inversion recovery sequence with a long TE, both the long T1 and the long T2 of pathologic abnormalities will contribute to the increased signal. In addition, the signal from surrounding fat is suppressed. Thus, STIR sequences will provide optimal contrast for most pathologic abnormalities.

STIR sequences suffer from lower S/N than conventional spin echo pulse sequences because of the suppression of the signal from all fat-containing structures. To compensate for this, most STIR sequences are performed using a narrow signal bandwidth (and increased sampling time, T_s). Typically, a bandwidth of ±4 or ±6 kHz is used, compared with the standard bandwidth of ±16 kHz for conventional spin echo sequences. In addition, the number of sections generated per unit time with STIR sequences is about one-half that of conventional T2-weighted sequences

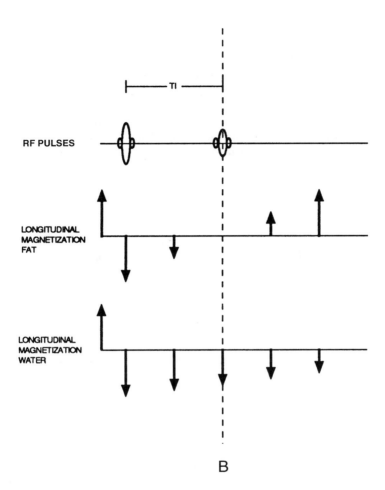

RF PULSES

LONGITUDINAL
MAGNETIZATION
FAT

LONGITUDINAL
MAGNETIZATION
WATER

B

FIGURE 11-24B. Fat recovers longitudinal magnetization much more rapidly than water. If a 180° pulse is followed by a 90° pulse at the time indicated by the dotted line, fat protons have essentially no longitudinal magnetization and therefore emit little signal.

for the same TR. This decrease of the number of sections compared with conventional spin echo sequences limits the routine use of conventional STIR sequences. As will be discussed below, by using a fast spin echo sequence, STIR images can be acquired much more rapidly, making their routine use practical.

3   FAST SPIN ECHO (FSE) IMAGING

Fast spin echo (FSE) sequences exploit the relationship of the strength of the phase-encoding gradient to the signal and spatial resolution of an image. To increase imaging speed, a different phase-encoding gradient strength can be used for each echo of a multiecho echo train following a 90° RF pulse. This increases the amount of phase-encoded data acquired per section per TR interval.

The FSE sequence acquires a train of up to 128 spin echoes (the actual number varies depending upon the particular imaging system and manufacturer) following each section selective 90° pulse. This is achieved by applying many 180° pulses in rapid succession to generate multiple spin echoes. A different phase-encoding gradient strength is used for each echo. The phase-encoding gradients are applied after each 180° pulse and then rewound prior to the next 180° pulse. The number of 180° pulses applied is referred to as the echo train length (ETL) and the spacing between echoes is referred to as the echo spacing (ESP). Thus, the FSE sequence acquires up to 128 lines of phase-encoded data for each section per TR interval before moving on to the next section. Therefore, for equal TR, phase matrix size, and NSA, the FSE sequence can reduce imaging time (compared with a conventional spin echo sequence) by a factor equal to ETL. The FSE pulse sequence diagram is shown in Figure 11-25.

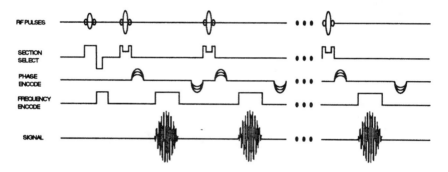

FIGURE 11-25.   FSE pulse diagram.

The fact that the phase-encoding gradients are rewound between 180° pulses of a FSE sequence is important. A phase-encoding gradient is applied after each 180° pulse and prior to the signal measurement. A gradient of equal magnitude but opposite direction is then applied after the signal measurement and prior to the next 180° pulse. The second gradient exactly cancels the phase changes induced by the phase-encoding gradient. Therefore, all of the phase changes induced by one phase-encoding gradient are canceled prior to the application of the next 180° pulse.

Why is this important? It is impossible to obtain perfect 180° pulses. Near the edges of a section, the 180° pulse will actually be less than 180° and therefore result in stimulated echoes in the tissue at the edges of a section. The stimulated echoes created by each 180° pulse will have their phase altered by the subsequent phase-encoding gradient. However, since new stimulated echoes are created by each subsequent 180° pulse, different stimulated echoes would experience different numbers of phase-encoding gradients.

For example, when using an ETL = 16, if the phase-encoding gradients were not rewound, the stimulated echo created by the first 180° pulse would experience all 16 phase-encoding gradients while the stimulated echo created by the last 180° pulse would experience only the last phase-encoding gradient. In order that the stimulated echoes from all of the 180° pulses remain in phase, the phase changes induced by the phase-encoding gradients must be eliminated between the 180° pulses. This is achieved by rewinding the phase-encoding gradients between 180° pulses. In fact, a large portion of the MR signal in an FSE image is sometimes derived from stimulated echoes (depending upon the echo spacing).

The method of data collection used for FSE sequences leads to unique imaging characteristics. Multiple echoes, each with a different TE and different phase-encoding gradient, are measured during each TR interval. The signals from all of these measurements are used to generate a single image. There is T2 decay of the MR signal between echoes of the multiecho train. Therefore, the early echoes have the most signal and the late echoes have the least signal, due to T2 decay. The signal loss for later echoes will therefore be greatest for tissue components with a short T2 value.

What about the effect of the different strength phase-encoding gradients? Phase-encoding gradients result in phase induced signal loss. The greater the strength of the phase-encoding gradient, the greater the degree of phase-induced signal loss. Therefore, those echoes acquired with the weaker phase-encoding gradients will have the least phase-induced signal loss and those echoes acquired with the stronger phase-encoding gradients will have the most phase-induced signal loss.

As noted in Chapter 8, echoes acquired with the weak phase-encoding gradients determine the signal and contrast of an image. These correspond to the low-frequency (and high-amplitude) sine and cosine functions of a Fourier series. Those echoes acquired with the strong phase-encoding gradients determine the spatial resolution and edge sharpness of an image. These correspond to the high-frequency (and low-amplitude) sine and cosine functions of a Fourier series.

What does all of this have to do with how contrast is determined for an FSE image? Suppose the weak phase-encoding gradients are applied to the late echoes of the multiecho train. This will cause the least amount of phase-induced signal loss for the late echoes. Since most of the signal and contrast of such an image will come from echoes with a long TE, the image will appear T2 weighted. The signal from these late echoes will be relatively enhanced because there is little phase gradient-induced signal loss. The term *relatively* here is meant compared with a conventional spin echo (CSE) sequence with an equivalent TE.

At the same time, the strong phase-encoding gradients are applied to the early echoes of each multiecho train. Echoes acquired with the strong phase-encoding gradients determine the spatial resolution and edge sharpness of the image. Since these are the earliest echoes, they will have the least amount of signal loss due to T2 decay. Therefore, the signal of the echoes that determine spatial resolution and edge sharpness will be relatively enhanced compared with a CSE sequence with an equivalent TE.

To review, then, T2-weighted FSE images are generated by applying the weak phase-encoding gradients to the late echoes and the strong phase-encoding gradients to the early echoes of the multiecho train of an FSE pulse sequence.

On the other hand, suppose the weak phase-encoding gradients are applied to the early echoes of each multiecho train. Since most of the signal and contrast of such an image will come from echoes with a short TE, the image will appear T1 weighted or proton density weighted depending upon the TR. At the same time, the strong phase-encoding gradients are applied to the late echoes of each multiecho train. The late echoes will therefore undergo significant signal loss due to both T2 decay and the signal loss induced by the strong phase-encoding gradients. These echoes will therefore have little useful residual signal. Since these echoes are necessary for spatial resolution and edge sharpness, the images will appear blurred, with structures having unsharp edges.

The blurring effect will be most pronounced for tissue with a short T2, since this tissue will have the greatest T2 decay for the late echoes. It is important to note that this edge blurring will be along the phase-encoding direction as a result of the method of phase encoded data collection for FSE images. The frequency-encoded data for FSE images is collected in the same manner as the frequency encoded data for CSE images. The edge blurring (and loss of spatial resolution) of T1-weighted and proton density weighted FSE images is most pronounced for small objects with a short T2 and thin objects oriented perpendicular to the phase-encoding direction. The degree of image blurring can be dramatic (Figure 11-26).

The choice of ETL and ESP will clearly affect the amount of blurring for T1-weighted and proton density weighted FSE images. Obviously blurring will be minimized for a shorter ETL and shorter ESP. In general, T1-weighted images are best acquired with CSE techniques. Since T1-weighted images use the earliest possible echo anyway, there is little advantage to using an FSE technique. The imaging time would be the same with both techniques to acquire the same number of sections. In rare instances where only a few sections are needed, the FSE technique might be advantageous.

If the FSE technique is used to generate T1-weighted or proton density weighted images, an ETL of 6 or less can be used to minimize image blurring. The minimum possible ESP should also be used. In addition, the use of a higher phase matrix will reduce blurring along the phase-encoding direction.

FSE images do not have a single TE time that can be specified. In general, when a TE (usually referred to as an effective TE) is chosen for an FSE sequence, the phase-encoding scheme is as follows: if the effective TE is chosen as $n \times ESP$, then the weakest phase-encoding gradients are applied to the n-th echo of each multiecho train ($n \leq ETL$). For example, suppose that ESP = 20 ms and ETL = 16. Then echoes will be collected at 20 ms, 40 ms, 60 ms, $\cdots$, 320 ms for each 16-echo multiecho train. If the phase matrix size is 192, then 12 such multiecho trains will be required (192/16 = 12). If an effective TE of 100 ms is chosen, then the 12 weakest phase-encoding gradients will be applied to the 5 th echo (5×20 ms = 100 ms) of each multiecho train.

What about the choice of TR for FSE sequences? For a given value of TR, phase matrix size, and NSA, the imaging time is inversely proportional to the ETL. However, the number of section locations is also inversely proportional to the ETL. It is advantageous to use as long a TR as possible, up to a point. The greater the TR value, the greater the degree of recovery of longitudinal magnetization between excitations and hence the greater the S/N of the image. In addition, the greater the value of TR, the greater the elimination of T1 weighting.

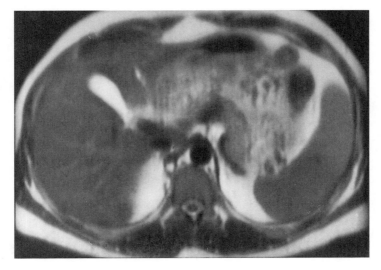

A

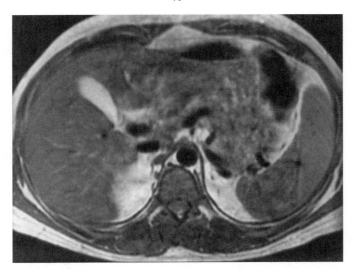

B

FIGURE 11-26 A&B. FSE proton density–weighted images through the mid abdomen. The image in (A) was obtained with an ETL of 64 and an effective TE of 17 ms. The image in (B) was obtained with an ETL of 4 and an effective TE of 17 ms. The blurring seen with the longer ETL is dramatic.

Beyond a certain point, however, there is little if any additional recovery of longitudinal magnetization as the TR is increased further. For most tissues, including water, there is near complete recovery of longitudinal magnetization for a TR value of about 6000 ms or greater. Therefore, there is little advantage (with respect to improving S/N and degree of T2 weighting) in using a TR of much greater than

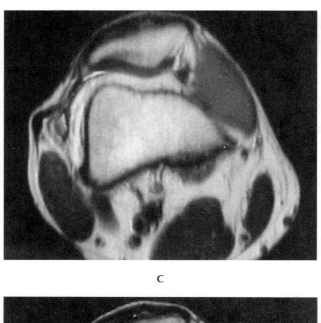

C

D

FIGURE 11-26 C&D.   FSE proton density–weighted images through the level of the mid-patellofemoral joint. The image in (C) was obtained with an ETL of 64 and an effective TE of 17 ms. The image in (D) was obtained with an ETL of 4 and an effective TE of 17 ms.

about 6000 ms . An exception is to use a higher TR in order to obtain a greater number of sections.

As the ETL is increased, echoes are acquired with later echo times. The later the echo time, the smaller the signal. This is most pronounced for tissues with a short T2. These tissues will have virtually no signal left for very late echoes. This loss of signal for late echoes will be most pronounced when the strong phase-encoding gradients are applied to the late echoes (e.g., for a proton density–weighted FSE image). This will increase the blurring of such images. This effect is negligible for T2-weighted FSE images since for these images the strong phase-encoding gradients are applied to the early echoes anyway.

When obtaining T2-weighted FSE images, a long effective TE must be chosen. The maximum value of the effective TE is directly proportional to the ETL (in fact, it is equal to the product of ETL and ESP). Therefore, the ETL must be chosen such that the desired effective TE can be attained. For example, suppose ESP = 20 ms and ETL = 4. Then the maximum achievable effective TE is 80 ms (4 × 20 ms = 80 ms). If an effective TE of 120 ms is desired, then an ETL of at least 6 would have to be used.

Ideally, then, assuming the ETL is long enough to attain the desired effective TE, the TR should be chosen to be about 6000 ms, and the ETL then adjusted accordingly to obtain the desired number of section locations.

What about the signal bandwidth (or sampling time, T_s)? The sampling time of each signal measurement is inversely proportional to the sampling rate. Therefore, by using a higher sampling rate, each phase-encoded signal can be measured more rapidly. For example, assuming that the signal bandwidth is equal to one-half of the sampling rate, the sampling time is equal to 8 ms when using a signal bandwidth of ±16 kHz, but the sampling time is equal to 4 ms when using a signal bandwidth of ±32 kHz. Thus, the ESP can be reduced by 4 ms when using a ±32-kHz signal bandwidth. The reduced ESP will reduce T2 decay between echoes and result in all echoes being acquired at earlier times. This will somewhat offset the loss of S/N associated with the higher signal bandwidth. The reduced ESP will also increase the number of section locations that can be acquired.

3.1 COUPLING OF SPINS

In general, the contrast characteristics of T2-weighted FSE images will be very similar to conventional spin echo T2-weighted images. One important exception is the appearance of lipids, such as subcutaneous fat. Depending upon the choice of parameters, the relative signal from lipids will be greater on FSE T2-weighted images than on conventional spin echo T2-weighted images. This effect can be explained using concepts from NMR spectroscopy.

Suppose that a sample containing protons is placed in an external magnetic field of strength 1.5 T. Then, expose the sample to RF radiation of varying frequency. The sample will absorb radiation at the resonance frequency of the protons within the sample. For pure water, this will occur at approximately 63.87 MHz. If the sample contained additional chemical species, then absorption would occur at additional frequencies. A plot of absorption versus frequency is the NMR spectrum of the sample.

Lipids within the human body contain long-chain fatty acids. Most of the protons within these molecules are contained in methyl (–CH₃), methylene (–CH₂), and methyne (–CH) groups. In a high-resolution NMR spectrum, the protons in each of these three groups have slightly different resonance frequencies when exposed to

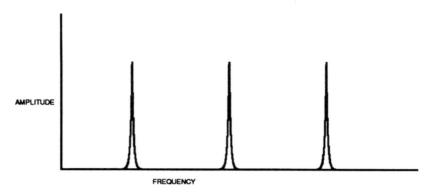

FIGURE 11-27. Graphical representation showing the expected NMR spectrum of long-chain fatty acids showing three peaks.

the same external magnetic field. This results from the fact that the local field experienced by each type of proton is slightly different due to their different chemical nature. One might therefore expect to see three different peaks within the NMR spectrum of long-chain fatty acids due to protons in each of these groups (Figure 11-27).

However, the signal emitted by each group is actually split into multiple closely spaced peaks. This splitting results from the interaction of protons on adjacent carbon atoms. How does this interaction come about? For example, at the end of a long-chain fatty acid, a methyl group and a methylene group are adjacent to one another ($-CH_2-CH_3$). Each of the two protons on the methylene group can assume one of two possible orientations with respect to the external field. That is, each of the two protons can be aligned with or against the external field. The alignment of each proton is independent.

Three distinct configurations of the two methylene protons are possible: both aligned with the field, both aligned against the field, or one aligned with and one aligned against the field. Each of these three configurations will result in a small but distinct change in the local magnetic field experienced by the methyl protons. Therefore, the observed NMR signal from the methyl protons is split into three peaks (Figure 11-28).

In an identical manner, the signal from the methylene protons will be split into four peaks by the three methyl protons (Figure 11-28). This results from the fact that there are four possible configurations of the three methyl protons with respect to the external field. Namely, all three aligned with the field, all three aligned against the field, two aligned with the field and one aligned against, and two aligned against the field and one aligned with the field.

Each peak in an NMR spectrum corresponds to a different resonance frequency. If the signal corresponding to the methyl protons is split into three peaks, this means that the methyl protons can precess at three closely spaced but different frequencies. At any instant of time, each individual proton precesses at a single frequency.

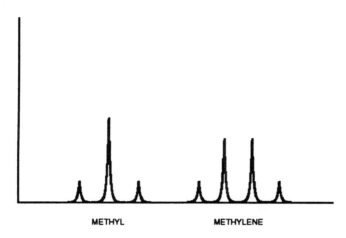

METHYL   METHYLENE

FIGURE 11-28. The signal from the methyl protons is split into three peaks, while the signal from the methylene protons is split into four peaks.

However, over time, as the configuration of the protons on adjacent carbon atoms changes, the precessional frequency of an individual proton will change.

The protons on the interacting groups are said to be coupled. A coupling constant, usually denoted by the letter J, is used as a measure of the splitting of the peak of one group of protons by another group to which they are coupled. Such **J couplings** are expressed in hertz and, unlike chemical shift differences (e.g., between water and lipid protons) they do not vary with the external magnetic field strength. This results from the fact that the local field changes that give rise to the coupling effects are derived from the intrinsic magnetic field of the protons. This intrinsic field is a result of the spin of the proton and is independent of the external main magnetic field.

A question that naturally arises is, why don't hydrogen atoms on the same carbon atom (in a long-chain fatty acid) or two hydrogen atoms on the same oxygen atom (in a water molecule) cause splitting of each other's peaks? Let's examine this by looking at the interaction of the two protons on a water molecule. Suppose that the external field B_0 is oriented along the z axis. Furthermore, suppose the oxygen atom of a water molecule is located at the origin of the coordinate system. Denote the two protons on the oxygen atom as H_A and H_B. Suppose the spatial orientation of the water molecule is fixed such that H_A is along the positive z axis and H_B is along the negative z axis.

Each proton acts as a tiny magnet. A magnet has a north pole and a south pole. Suppose that at a particular instant of time, H_A is oriented such that its north pole points along the B_0 field. Then, H_B will be closer to the south pole of H_A (Figure 11-29A). On the other hand, suppose that at a different point in time, H_A is oriented such that its south pole points along the B_0 field. In this case, H_B will be closer to the north pole of H_A (Figure 11-29B). It therefore seems that the local field experienced by H_B is dependent upon the orientation of the field of the proton H_A. However, this argument assumes that the spatial orientation of the water molecule itself is fixed.

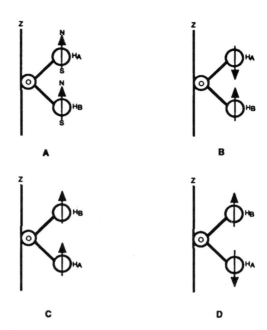

FIGURE 11-29. Hydrogen atoms attached to the same carbon atom do not cause splitting due to the rapid motion of the water molecules.

Suppose the spatial orientation of the water molecule is reversed such that H_A is on the negative z axis and H_B is on the positive z axis. In this case, when H_A is oriented with its north pole pointing along the B_0 field, then H_B will be closer to the north pole of H_A (Figure 11-29C). Likewise, when H_A is oriented with its south pole along the B_0 field, then H_B will be closer to the south pole of H_A (Figure 11-29D). This is the exact reverse of the situation above. Therefore, the local field experienced by the protons on a water molecule is also dependent upon the spatial orientation of the water molecule itself.

Because of the rapid tumbling motion of water molecules in solution, the relative orientation of the two protons in space is constantly changing. This causes the local field at H_B to be independent of the orientation of the field of H_A (and vice versa). Therefore, these protons do not cause splitting of the NMR peak of their neighbor. In essence, due to the rapid tumbling motion of the water molecules, each proton experiences an average local field (i.e., averaged over all possible orientations of the water molecule in space). If the tumbling motion were not rapid, then this averaging effect would not occur.

An identical argument applies to hydrogen atoms attached to the same carbon atom. Due to the rapid rotation around carbon–carbon bonds, there is an averaging of the local field experienced by an individual proton due to its neighbor. Such protons that are bonded to the same atom and do not cause splitting of each other's peaks are usually referred to as equivalent protons.

Since the orientation of each proton with respect to B_0 also changes in time, why isn't there a similar averaging effect on the field experienced by protons on adjacent carbon atoms? Although there is a constant exchange between orientations of individual protons with respect to the external field B_0 (i.e., alignment with or against the external field), this exchange is relatively slow. It is many orders of magnitude slower than the tumbling rate of water molecules in solution. In fact, the rate of this exchange is dependent upon T1 relaxation. In general, the T1 relaxation rate of biologic tissues is not rapid enough to prevent splitting of the peaks.

What does all of this have to do with the MR signal of fat on FSE T2-weighted images? The T1 value of lipid protons is on the order of 100 ms. It can be shown mathematically that if T1 = 100 ms, then approximately every 70 ms (70 = 100 × ln2, where ln is the natural logarithm) about half of the protons will have changed their alignment with respect to the external field at least once. Some will have changed their alignment many times.

Each time a proton changes its alignment, the field experienced by other protons to which it is coupled also changes. These local field changes result in dephasing of protons on adjacent carbon atoms. This is equivalent to T2 decay. 180° pulses will compensate for fixed local field differences. Fixed means that the field differences remain constant over the interval of application of the 180° pulse and subsequent signal measurement (i.e., over the interval TE).

When conventional spin echo T2-weighted images are acquired, a long TE is used. As a result, coupled protons will undergo one or more local field changes during the interval TE. These field changes are therefore not fixed and are not compensated for by the 180° pulse. This lowers the T2 value of lipid protons. If, on the other hand, the 180° pulses are very closely spaced, then the local field changes will essentially remain unchanged between 180° pulses. Under this circumstance, the local field changes caused by adjacent protons will not induce dephasing. In essence, the application of closely spaced 180° pulses decouples coupled protons and therefore prevents dephasing.

When FSE T2-weighted images are acquired, many closely spaced 180° pulses are used. This results in decoupling of the lipid protons which causes their signal to be relatively increased. The closely spaced 180° pulses of an FSE sequence cause the T2 value of lipid protons to increase. This accounts for the relatively increased signal of lipid-containing structures on FSE images compared with conventional spin echo images.

A simple means of reducing the lipid signal on fast spin echo sequences is to delay the application of the first 180° pulse following a 90° pulse. Over the interval of the time delay, coupled protons will undergo one or more local field changes. These field changes will not be compensated for by the first 180° pulse. This will result in some T2 decay and therefore lower the signal of the lipid protons. If there is a delay only prior to the first 180° pulse, it will add minimal additional imaging time to the sequence.

4   ECHOPLANAR IMAGING

As described in the section on FSE imaging, the FSE sequence reduces imaging time by acquiring multiple phase samples (up to 128) per TR interval. In fact, the fastest possible imaging sequence would acquire all phase samples following a single excitation. In addition to a reduction of imaging time, there are other advantages to such an imaging scheme. If only a single excitation is used, then at the time of the excitation there is maximal longitudinal magnetization. With conventional multiexcitation sequences, there is never complete recovery of longitudinal magnetization by all tissues between excitations. Acquiring all of the phase-encoded data following a single excitation is equivalent to using a very long TR (essentially an infinite TR).

What are some of the difficulties with implementing such a sequence? Immediately following an excitation, the MR signal will be maximal. However, the signal will then rapidly decay. Once the signal decays beyond a certain point, no useful signal measurements can be obtained. Therefore, if all of the phase-encoded signal measurements are to be made following a single excitation, this process must be completed prior to such decay. For conventional spin echo sequences, the signal decays by a factor of $e^{-t/T2}$ at t milliseconds after an excitation.

For GRE sequences, the signal decays by a factor of $e^{-t/T2^*}$ at t ms after an excitation. For all tissues, T2* < T2, which means that the decay of signal on GRE sequences is always faster than the decay of spin echo signals. These factors ignore the signal decay due to the phase-encoding gradients themselves, which induce additional signal loss due to dephasing.

For most biologic tissues (with the exception of pure water), T2 is on the order of 100 ms or less (with T2* being lower in value). Even assuming a T2 (or T2*) value of 100 ms, the signal will decay by a factor of $e^{-3} = 0.05$ even 300 ms after excitation. This means that for a tissue with a T2 value of 100 ms, only 5% of the signal will remain 300 ms after excitation. This does not take into account the signal loss associated with the phase-encoding gradients. Therefore, for most tissues, all of the signal measurements must be obtained within at most several hundred milliseconds of excitation in order that there be useful signal to measure.

What is the minimum spacing between echoes that can be achieved using spin echoes? Spin echoes require 180° pulses. In order to apply a 180° pulse, a section selective gradient must be turned on, the 180° pulse applied, and the section selective gradient then turned off. It takes a minimum of about 5–7 ms to accomplish all of these steps. Therefore, even if nothing else needed to be done, the minimum spacing between 180° pulses is about 5–7 ms.

In addition to application of the 180° pulses, signal measurements must be performed following each 180° pulse. This would add an additional amount of time to the spacing between echoes. Even if this were ignored, the minimum echo spacing (for spin echoes) would still be about 5–7 ms. Suppose a 128-phase matrix is used. Since 128×7 ms = 896 ms, using multiple spin echoes following a single excitation, most of the signal measurements would have to be made 400 ms or more following excitation. These late signal measurements would have little useful signal.

What is the minimum spacing between echoes that can be achieved using gradient echoes? Gradient echoes are created by using a bilobed gradient. The first lobe (or rephasing lobe) is of equal magnitude, opposite direction, and one-half the duration of the second lobe. The second lobe serves as the read gradient for signal measurement. The minimum spacing between gradient echoes is therefore equal to at least 1.5 times the duration of the read gradient. The read gradient duration equals the time of signal measurement.

The time required for the signal measurement process is equal to the reciprocal of the sampling rate multiplied by the number of signal samples. The sampling rate is typically equal to twice the signal bandwidth. When 256 frequency samples are used and the signal bandwidth is ±16 kHz, the signal measurement process takes 8 ms. This can be dramatically shortened by use of a higher signal bandwidth. If, for example, the signal bandwidth were ±256 kHz, the signal measurement process for 256 frequency samples would be equal to 0.5 ms. However, there is a penalty for using such a high signal bandwidth.

In order to use an increased signal bandwidth, the strength of the read gradient must be increased accordingly. If, for example, the FOV is 40 cm and the signal bandwidth is ±16 kHz, then the frequency gradient across the FOV is 32 kHz/40 cm, which equals 800 Hz/cm. In order to convert this to field strength per centimeter, recall that at a field strength of 1.5 T (which equals 15,000 G), the precessional frequency of protons is 63.87 MHz. This corresponds to $15,000 \, G/(63.87 \times 10^6 \, Hz)$, which equals approximately 0.00024 G/Hz. Therefore, 800 Hz/cm corresponds to a magnetic field gradient of approximately 800×0.00024 G/cm, which equals 0.2 G/cm.

If a signal bandwidth of strength ±256 kHz were used, this would require a read gredient strength of $(512/32) \times (0.2 \, G/cm)$, which is 3.2 G/cm. The standard gradient coils used on most imaging systems can achieve a gradient of only about 1.5 G/cm. In addition, if the FOV is decreased, the gradient strength must be increased proportionately. For example, to achieve a 20-cm FOV with a signal bandwidth of ±256 kHz would require a read gradient strength of 6.4 G/cm. Therefore, in order to use very high signal bandwidths, specialized gradient coils must be used and even then, the achievable FOV is limited.

Suppose a single 90° excitation pulse is applied to a sample of protons. In addition, suppose a bilobed frequency-encoding gradient is rapidly turned on and off and that signal measurements are made during the second lobe. If the read gradient strength is such that the signal bandwidth is ±256 kHz, and if a 256-frequency matrix size is used, then the time required to perform each signal measurement is about 0.5 ms . If the desired phase matrix size is 64, then the time required to complete all of the signal measurements is 32 ms . If the desired phase matrix size is 128, then the time required to complete all of the signal measurements is 64 ms

When such a series of gradient echoes is acquired following a single excitation, it is referred to as an **echoplanar** imaging sequence. How is the signal in an echoplanar imaging sequence phase encoded?

A strong negative phase-encoding gradient is applied prior to the first signal measurement. Suppose this gradient is of strength –G. If 128 phase-encoding steps are used, then each subsequent phase-encoding gradient is of strength +G/64. For the first signal measurement, the net gradient will be –G + (G/64). For the second signal measurement, the net gradient will be –G + (2G/64). For the n-th signal measurement, the net gradient will be –G + (nG/64). Therefore, for the last signal measurement, the net gradient will be –G + (128G/64) = +G. In this way, the phase encoding will be incrementally stepped from negative gradients to positive gradients in sequential fashion.

Since the phase is incremented in very small increments between phase-encoding steps, this technique is sometimes referred to as "blip" echoplanar imaging. The "blip" refers to the small phase changes. The phase-encoding gradients are turned on during the first lobe (i.e., the rephasing lobe) of each frequency-encoding gradient. No signal measurements are being performed during this time. Therefore, the phase-encoding does not add time to the imaging sequence.

In order to avoid aliasing along the phase direction, the phase-encoded gradient strength must be chosen such that the highest phase component of the signal advances through at most one-half cycle between signal measurements. For example, if a 128-phase matrix is used and the total time of the signal measurement process is 64 ms, then the sampling rate along the phase-encoding direction is 128 samples per 64 ms = 2 samples per millisecond = 2000 samples per second. This corresponds to a sampling rate of 2 kHz.

Since the size of the phase matrix is 128, this corresponds to a phase change of (2000/128) Hz per pixel, which is equal to 15.6 Hz per pixel. At 1.5 T, the difference in precessional frequency between lipid and water protons is approximately 220 Hz. Since 220/15.6 is approximately 14, the positional misregistration of lipid protons along the phase-encoding direction is over a distance of 14 pixels. This results in severe chemical shift artifact along the phase-encoding direction. Some commercially available imaging systems implement echoplanar imaging using excitation pulses that are both section selective and chemically selective in order to excite only water protons in each section. This is an effective means of suppressing the signal from lipid protons on echoplanar images and will therefore reduce chemical shift artifact.

The above scheme for performing echoplanar imaging obtains all signal measurements following a single excitation using many gradient echoes. The images will therefore be T2* weighted. More T2 weighting can be obtained in the following sequence: Start with a 90° pulse followed at time TE/2 by a 180° pulse so that a spin echo occurs at time TE. The gradient echo measurements can then be performed so that the group of measurements are centered on the spin echo. This means that half of the signal measurements are performed prior to the time TE and half of the signal measurements are performed after the time TE. In addition, the weakest phase-encoding gradients are obtained around the center of the spin echo. In an identical manner as that with phase-encoding of fast spin echo sequences, this means that the effective echo time will be TE. With such an implementation, the signal measurements are centered around a spin echo (Figure 11-30). Even though each of the individual signal measurements are from gradient echoes, since the maximal signal occurs at TE (the center of a spin echo), the overall signal will be relatively T2 weighted rather than T2* weighted.

To summarize, then, the echoplanar imaging method is the fastest possible means of generating an MR image. It works by performing all phase-encoded signal measurements following a single excitation. It uses a very strong frequency-encoding gradient in order to perform all signal measurements prior to complete loss of useful signal. This is equivalent to a very large signal bandwidth. Since the S/N is inversely

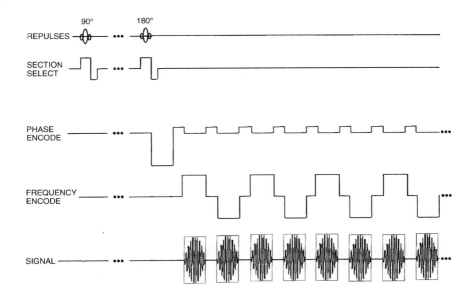

FIGURE 11-30.   Echoplanar pulse diagram.

proportional to the square root of the signal bandwidth, this results in a significant decrease of the S/N. For example, compared with a standard signal bandwidth of ±16 kHz, use of a signal bandwidth of ±256 kHz will diminish the S/N by a factor of √(16/256), which equals approximately 4. This is somewhat offset by the use of an essentially infinite TR.

12 Multicoils

For a given imaging region, S/N is maximized by placing the receiver coil as close as possible to the region of interest. The coil diameter should be equal to the distance from the region of interest to the coil. In general, this is achieved by a surface coil, provided that the region of interest is small (and therefore a small FOV can be used). For large regions of interest, it is not practical (or optimal) to use a single surface coil.

In regions close to the coil, surface coils provide markedly improved S/N, compared to body coils. Surface coils are used as receive-only, with the excitation pulse provided by the body coil. The sensitive region of a surface coil is severely limited, typically on the order of the coil diameter. If an object is located within the sensitive region, then it will be in close proximity to the coil and therefore have a high signal.

On the other hand, the noise received by a coil is also limited to noise originating in the sensitive region. The total noise in an image ordinarily comes from the entire object being imaged. However, when using a surface coil, only noise originating within the very limited sensitive region of the coil will be of significant amplitude. This markedly reduces the noise within the image, and hence the significant improvement in S/N of a surface coil.

When used individually, surface coils can provide only small FOV images. Suppose that multiple surface coils are used simultaneously. The phase of the signal in each coil will depend upon the coil orientation. This is similar to the situation when using a quadrature coil. Recall that a quadrature coil consists of two coils oriented at 90° with respect to one another. The signals in the two coils are therefore 90° out of phase. Prior to being fed into the receiver circuit, the signal in one of the coils is phase shifted back by 90°. The two signals are then added together and fed into a single circuit. The process of phase shifting the two signals prior to their being added will be error free provided that the exact difference in orientation of the two coils is known.

Suppose several surface coils are used simultaneously in a receive-only mode. Unless the exact orientations of the coils is fixed and known, addition of the signals into a single circuit will result in signal loss due to phase differences between the signals. However, suppose the signal from each coil is separately fed into its own receiver channel and that the k space data from each coil is analyzed separately to reconstruct an image. Each individual image will be identical to the image that would have been obtained had the coil been used by itself. Each image will therefore have a relatively small effective FOV.

A composite image can be formed by adding the individual images in each coil. By adding the individual images (rather than the individual signals themselves) we have eliminated the need to know the exact phase relationship of the signals. The addition of the individual images is done on a pixel-by-pixel basis. The effective

FOV of the composite image will essentially equal the region spanned by all of the individual coils. This FOV is obviously greater than the effective FOV of the individual surface coils. Therefore, the composite image will have the S/N of a surface coil but the effective FOV of a much larger coil.

Such an arrangement of individual surface coils acting independently and simultaneously in a receive-only mode is referred to as a **multicoil** (or sometimes, a phased-array coil). On a practical basis, the number of individual coils that can be used as a multicoil is limited by the fact that each coil requires its own receiver electronics. Such hardware is very expensive. At present, multicoils are available with a maximum of four separate coils.

There are a number of different ways to combine the individual images into a composite image. Let P_{ic} be the intensity of the i-th pixel in the composite image. Let P_{in} be the intensity of the i-th pixel in the image of coil n, for n = 1, 2, 3, and 4. Perhaps the simplest method is to let the signal intensity of each pixel in the composite image equal the square root of the sum of the squares of corresponding pixel values in the individual coil images. That is, $P_{ic} = \sqrt{[(P_{i1})^2 + (P_{i2})^2 + (P_{i3})^2 + (P_{i4})^2]}$. This method is referred to as the sum of the squares technique.

More complicated methods would weight the contribution from each coil to a given pixel in the composite image based upon the proximity of the pixel to each coil. For example, suppose a pixel is located within the effective FOV of coil 3. Then it would make the most sense to use largely the signal from coil 3 to represent such pixels in the composite image.

In addition, for pixels located within the effective FOV of a given coil, the closer the pixel is to the coil, the greater its relative signal will be. Recall that when using a surface coil, signal in structures right next to the coil (such as subcutaneous fat) will be markedly increased. It therefore makes the most sense to weight the signal within the effective FOV of a given coil so that the weighting is inversely related to the distance from the coil. This way, structures located right next to the coil will not have such markedly increased signal. This would make the image more uniform.

What is the effect of using a weighting technique on ghost artifact? Suppose respiratory motion of the subcutaneous fat beneath one of the coils gives rise to ghost artifact. Ordinarily, the ghosts would appear as curvilinear lines of signal, shaped like the moving structure from which they arise. Since the ghosts arise from the very-high-signal subcutaneous fat, even ghosts far from the coil would still have substantial signal. In fact, the ghosts arising from structures next to one coil might be placed within the effective FOV of the other coils. If no weighting is used, then ghosts arising from structures beneath one coil would be displayed throughout the entire image. However, if inverse weighting is used, the ghosts would only be displayed within the effective FOV of the coil nearest the structure from which they arise.

Since the sum of squares technique is the simplest recombination algorithm, it is the technique most commonly employed. When this technique is used, structures located near the coils will have markedly increased signal in the composite image. Therefore, subcutaneous fat will have greatly increased signal even on T2 weighted images. In addition, phase ghost artifact will be propagated through the entire image since no weighting is used.

The improvement in S/N of a multicoil compared with a body coil is substantial. There is an approximately two-fold improvement in S/N for structures located near the center of the coil array. This results from the fact that N independent coils will provide an improvement in S/N of $\sqrt{N}$. For structures located near the individual coils, the improvement in S/N is substantially greater.

Most multicoils used in body imaging consist of two adjacent anterior coils and two adjacent posterior coils. Most multicoils used in spine imaging consist of four to six adjacent coils along a straight line. Depending upon the portion of the spine being imaged, only four of the coils are used at any one time.

One final point relating to multicoils should be mentioned. When a coil is receiving a signal, a current will be flowing through the coil. This current will have an associated magnetic field. If two such coils are in close proximity, then the magnetic field associated with current flow in one coil can itself induce a current in the other coil (and vice versa). This is referred to as induction. The magnitude of the induced current in an adjacent coil is dependent upon the distance between the coils, the size and shape of the coils, and the size of the currents flowing in the coils.

If two adjacent coils are overlapped by the proper amount, their mutual inductance can be made to be zero. In fact, the pair of anterior coils and the pair of posterior coils in a pelvic multicoil array are typically overlapped by a small amount such that their mutual inductance is zero.

13 Vascular MRI

In order to generate vascular MR images without the use of intravascular contrast agents, one of two techniques is currently employed: time-of-flight (TOF) angiography or phase contrast (PC) angiography. These techniques of MR angiography (MRA) rely on entirely different principles to generate vascular images. They will therefore be described separately.

1 TIME-OF-FLIGHT MRA

1.1 FLOW-RELATED SIGNAL LOSS

Suppose a blood vessel courses through a section of tissue. Depending upon the flow velocity, the blood may remain in the section for only a short period of time. When performing conventional spin echo pulse sequences, the time between the application of the 90° pulse and the 180° pulse is TE/2. Both of these pulses are section selective and will only excite tissue within the single section. Therefore, if the protons within a blood vessel flow out of the section between the time of the 90° and 180° pulses, these protons will not be refocused by the refocusing 180° pulse.

At the same time, the new protons that have moved into a section after the 90° pulse will have no net transverse magnetization. The effect of a 180° pulse on these protons will therefore be to invert their longitudinal magnetization, without creating transverse magnetization. Such protons will not emit a signal. If all of the protons within a blood vessel move out of the excited section between the 90° and the 180° pulses, there will be no net signal emitted from the vessel. This results in intravascular **signal void**. This effect is usually referred to as flow-related signal loss (Figure 13-1).

If blood is flowing at velocity V, then the distance it travels in time TE/2 is equal to V × TE/2. If this distance exceeds the thickness of the section being imaged, then there will be an intravascular signal void. This assumes that the direction of flowing blood is perpendicular to the section. When the blood flow is oriented at an angle θ with respect to the plane of the section, signal void will occur when Vsinθ × (TE/2) exceeds the section thickness.

In general, then, when performing conventional spin echo images, the degree of intravascular signal loss due to TOF effects is dependent upon the ratio (Vsinθ × TE)/(section thickness). When this ratio is greater than 1, an intravascular signal void will occur. This is the case for most arterial flow (unless the flow is parallel or near parallel to the plane of section, in which case sinθ is close to 0). When this ratio is significantly less than 1, TOF effects will not result in intravascular signal void. For such cases, one can alter the imaging parameters to maximize flow-related signal loss (if desired). This is achieved by using thinner sections and longer TE

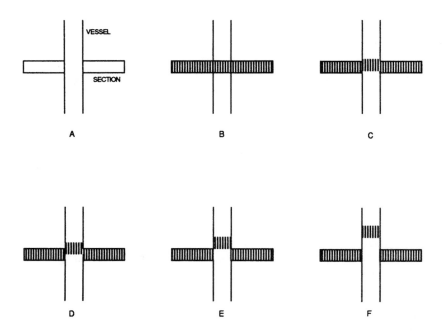

FIGURE 13-1. In (A), a vessel is seen coursing through a section of tissue. In (B), the entire section, including the portion of the vessel within the section, is excited by an RF pulse. The excited tissue is shown by the cross-hatched area. In (C–F), the excited protons within the vessel progressively move further downstream from the section. In (E), all of the excited protons within the vessel have just moved completely out of the section.

and choosing the plane of section as perpendicular as possible to the direction of flow in the vessel of interest.

Saturation pulses can be used to selectively eliminate the signal from arterial and/or venous blood. For any given section, arterial blood and venous blood will usually flow in opposite directions. By applying saturation pulses selectively to the venous and/or arterial in-flow side of a section, selective saturation of venous and/or arterial blood is accomplished (Figure 13-2). When performing multisection imaging, saturation pulses are most effective for sections located at either end of the imaging volume. This results from the fact that the end sections of the imaging volume are closest to the tissue exposed to the saturation pulses (Figure 13-3). For very slow venous flow, saturation pulses will be ineffective.

Flow-related signal loss and/or saturation pulses can therefore be used to generate images where soft tissue structures will have signal and vascular structures will appear as relative signal voids. This is sometimes referred to as "black-blood" imaging.

1.2 FLOW-RELATED ENHANCEMENT

Suppose the flow within a given vessel is such that $(V\sin\theta \times TE)/(\text{section thickness})$ is much less than 1. Then when using conventional spin echo sequences, only a

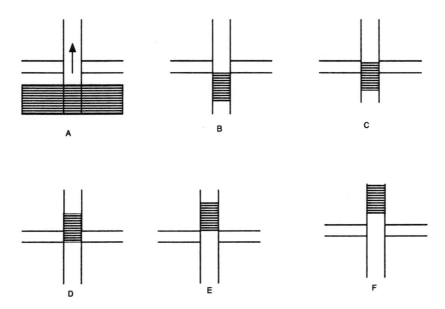

FIGURE 13-2. In (A), a vessel courses through a section of tissue with flow direction as shown. A large saturation pulse is placed on the in-flow side of the section which includes the portion of the vessel leading into the section. All tissue excited by the saturation pulse is shown in the cross-hatched region. In (B), the excited protons within the vessel have moved toward the section. In (C) and (D), protons within the blood vessel have been previously excited by the saturation pulse. If an excitation pulse is applied to the section, the protons within the vessel will essentially emit no signal. In (E) and (F), the protons in the blood vessel previously excited by the saturation pulse have moved beyond the section. If an excitation pulse is applied to the section now, the protons within the vessel will emit signal.

small portion of the intravascular protons within a section move out of the section between application of the 90° and 180° pulses. This will result in significant intravascular signal. The shorter the TE and the thicker the section, the greater this effect will be.

On the other hand, suppose the flow within a vessel is such that (Vsinθ × TE)/(section thickness) is much less than 1 and (Vsinθ × TR)/(section thickness) is greater than 1. This means that only a small portion of the intravascular protons move out of the section between the 90° and 180° pulses (i.e., over the interval of time TE/2), but that all of the intravascular protons move out of the section between successive 90° pulses (i.e., over the interval of time TR). Therefore, all of the intravascular protons will be replaced by protons from outside of the section between successive 90° pulses. Since these protons will not have been previously excited, they will have maximal longitudinal magnetization. This is equivalent to all of the intravascular protons undergoing complete T1 relaxation between successive 90° pulses. This results in even greater signal from intravascular protons. The replacement of previously excited intravascular protons by previously unexcited intravascular protons is sometimes referred to as replenishment.

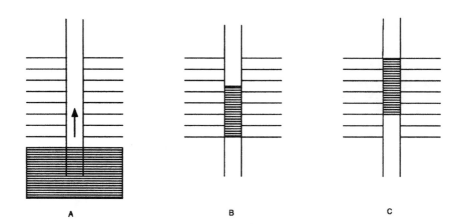

FIGURE 13-3. In (A), a vessel courses through multiple sections with flow in the direction indicated. A large saturation pulse is placed on the in-flow side of the section which includes the portion of the vessel leading into the section. In (B), the protons in the blood vessel previously excited by the saturation pulse have moved into the sections on the in-flow side of the vessel. In (C), the previously excited protons have moved into the sections on the out-flow side of the vessel.

Thus, the combined effect of (Vsinθ × TE)/(section thickness) being much less than 1 and (Vsinθ × TR)/(section thickness) being greater than 1 is to increase intravascular signal. This is referred to as **flow-related enhancement**. Flow-related enhancement can therefore be used to generate images where soft tissue structures will have low signal and vascular structures will appear bright. This is sometimes referred to as "bright-blood" imaging.

In order to maximize vessel/background contrast, the imaging parameters should be chosen to maximize vessel signal and minimize background signal. As noted above, vessel signal is maximized by using the shortest possible TE, relatively thick sections, and a TR such that (Vsinθ × TR)/(section thickness) ≥1.

To minimize the signal from nonvascular structures, it would be optimal to choose TR such that (Vsinθ × TR)/(section thickness) = 1 (i.e., choose TR as short as possible such that there is still complete replacement of intravascular protons with previously unexcited protons between excitations). As TR is shortened, the time for recovery of longitudinal magnetization in nonvascular structures (i.e., stationary structures) is minimized. This reduces the signal in these structures.

Therefore, to optimize vessel/background contrast, one should use the shortest possible TE and choose TR only as long as necessary to allow complete replenishment of the intravascular protons between excitations. However, there is an additional reason for using the shortest possible TE to maximize vessel/background contrast. This is an important point and will now be discussed in some detail.

Flow (or motion) in the presence of gradients results in phase-induced signal loss. It has been previously shown that for constant velocity (V) motion, the phase change (Δφ) induced by a gradient of strength G, applied over a time t is proportional to GVt^2. Likewise, for motion with constant acceleration, the phase change is proportional to t^3. In fact, it can be shown that for motion of order n (n = 0 corresponds to no motion, n = 1 corresponds to constant velocity motion, n = 2 correspond to constant acceleration motion, etc.), the phase change is proportional to $t^{(n+1)}$. Motion of higher order than constant acceleration is usually referred to as "jerk."

Therefore, the phase changes induced by the section select and read gradients will result in intravascular phase-induced signal loss. Recall that flow compensation techniques can eliminate phase-induced signal loss from constant velocity motion (by using multilobed gradients). However, it is very difficult to compensate for phase-induced signal loss from higher order motion. Unfortunately, the motion of flowing blood is rather complex and is not accurately represented by constant velocity motion. Higher order motion is also present. It is for this reason that it is important to use the shortest possible TE to minimize phase-induced intravascular signal loss.

The minimum TE that can be achieved with conventional spin echo sequences is significantly greater than that which can be achieved with GRE sequences. Thus, GRE sequences will usually provide greater flow-related enhancement compared with conventional spin echo sequences. GRE sequences with the shortest possible TE and relatively short TR will usually provide optimal vessel-to-background contrast.

The effect of flip angle on vessel-to-background contrast is somewhat more complex. In general, the larger the flip angle, the less the recovery of longitudinal magnetization in stationary tissues between excitation pulses for a given TR. Therefore, in general, the greater the flip angle (up to 90°) the lower the signal from stationary tissue.

If the flow within a vessel is such that there is complete replacement of protons between excitations, then a 90° pulse will provide maximal vascular signal. However, if there is not complete replenishment of intravascular protons between excitations, then a steady state will be established for those intravascular protons that are not replaced by fresh protons. These protons behave as stationary tissue (at least for the few excitations for which they remain within the excited plane of section). Therefore, the maximal signal from such protons will not necessarily occur for 90° pulses. Hence, for very slow flow (i.e., flow that results in little replenishment of protons between excitations) a less than 90° pulse may provide optimal signal.

If multisection imaging is performed, the effect of flow-related enhancement is more complex. Suppose the arterial flow in two adjacent sections (labeled section 1 and section 2) is being imaged. In addition, suppose the direction of arterial flow is from section 1 to section 2. Following excitation of section 1, some arterial intravascular protons from section 1 will move into section 2 prior to excitation of section 2. These protons will have diminished longitudinal magnetization, as well as some residual transverse magnetization. These protons will contribute less than maximal signal following excitation of section 2. This will diminish the intravascular signal from arteries in section 2 compared with the signal that would otherwise be emitted had section 1 not been previously excited. This effect is more significant as more sections are excited during each TR interval.

Suppose a volume acquisition is performed. Let the volume be of length L and consist of s sections each of thickness T (i.e., L = sT). Suppose a vessel crosses perpendicular to the volume with flow of velocity V. During the TR interval, fresh protons will travel into the volume to a depth equal to V × TR. If V × TR ≥ sT, then fresh intravascular protons will completely replace all of the previously excited protons within the volume. If V × TR = nT, where n < s, then only the first n sections of the volume will have their intravascular protons completely replenished between excitations.

Therefore, flow-related enhancement will be most prominent at the in-flow (or end) sections of a volume acquisition. Arterial flow-related enhancement will be maximal at the arterial in-flow end of the volume and venous flow-related enhancement will be maximal at the venous in-flow end of the volume. As one goes deeper into the imaging volume, the replacement of previously excited intravascular protons by fresh protons between excitations will become less and less (depending upon the velocity of vascular flow). This effect is sometimes referred to as entry slice phenomenon. That is, flow-related enhancement will be greatest at the entry side of a volume.

In addition to the above effect, when saturation pulses are used to selectively suppress arterial or venous signal, the closer the saturation pulses are to the section of interest the more effective the saturation pulses will be. When performing multisection imaging, saturation pulses can be applied only at the ends of the imaging volume (the volume being the "stack" of multiple sections) at the beginning of each TR interval. Therefore, as more sections are included during each TR interval, those sections furthest from the in-flow end of arterial (or venous) signal will be less affected by the saturation pulses.

As a result of the entry slice phenomenon and effect of the proximity of saturation pulses, single section acquisitions are the most effective means of producing TOF bright-blood vascular images.

When performing TOF MRA, saturation pulses can be used to determine direction of flow. Suppose a saturation pulse is applied within the FOV perpendicular to a vessel (Figure 10-17). Stationary tissue exposed to the saturation pulse will emit no signal. This will appear as a black band across stationary tissue exposed to the saturation pulse. However, since there is a finite time delay between application of the saturation pulse (and its accompanying spoiler gradients) and the following excitation pulse, some blood will flow into the saturation band during this time delay. This will result in some signal within the vessel (within the saturation band) at the in-flow side of the vessel. The depth of penetration of this signal is dependent upon the flow velocity.

2   PHASE CONTRAST MRA

PC techniques rely upon gradient-induced phase changes between stationary spins and moving spins. The PC technique relies on the difference in the effect of a magnetic field gradient on stationary and moving protons. These effects have been previously discussed in the section on flow compensation techniques but will be reviewed in the context of PC techniques.

Suppose a linear gradient is applied along the z axis such that the magnetic field strength at any point, denoted by B(x,y,z), is given by B(x,y,z) = $(B_0 + z\Delta B)$, where ΔB is a constant. Before the gradient is turned on, all (transverse magnetization) M_T

will precess at the same frequency, γB_0, where γ is the gyromagnetic ratio. While the gradient is on, M_T at the point (x,y,z) will precess at frequency $\gamma(B_0 + z\Delta B)$. Once the gradient is turned off, all M_T will once again precess at the same frequency, γB_0. While the gradient is on, M_T in different voxels will precess at different frequencies and will no longer remain in phase. Therefore, the effect of a transient gradient is to alter the phase relationship of M_T as a function of position.

Phase is a relative quantity that must be defined with respect to a reference. In this discussion, we will use as our reference, stationary tissue located at the origin (0,0,0). Since z = 0 at the origin, even while the gradient is on, the field strength at the origin does not change because it is given by $(B_0 + 0\Delta B) = B_0$. Hence, M_T located at the origin will precess at the same (resonance) frequency before, during, and after the gradient is turned on.

Suppose stationary tissue is located at the point (x,y,z). If the gradient is turned on for a period of time T, then M_T at this point will undergo a phase change of magnitude $\gamma\Delta BzT$ cycles. If $\gamma\Delta BzT = n + \phi$, where n is an integer, and $\phi < 1$, then the actual phase change is equal to ϕ cycles. That is, a phase change of an integral number of cycles does not alter the phase; only a change of a fraction of a cycle alters the phase.

Suppose a blood vessel is oriented along the z axis and has flow in the positive z direction at constant velocity V. Then M_T within the blood vessel will change its position while the gradient is on and therefore change its precessional frequency. Suppose M_T within the vessel is located at the point (x,y,z) at time t = 0 when the gradient is turned on. Then at time t = T, it will be located at the point (x,y,z+VT). For all times t in between (i.e., 0 < t < T), it will be located at the point (x,y,z+Vt). What is the total phase change that M_T will experience from t = 0 to t = T. It has been previously shown in Chapter 10 that the total phase change will be equal to $[\gamma\Delta BzT + (1/2)\gamma V\Delta BT^2]$.

Therefore, if a linear gradient of the form $B(x,y,z) = (B_0 + z\Delta B)$ is applied, for a time T,

1. For stationary tissue, this will induce a phase change of magnitude $\gamma\Delta BzT$.
2. For tissue moving at constant velocity V along the direction of the gradient, this will induce a phase change of magnitude $[\gamma\Delta BzT + (1/2)\gamma V\Delta BT^2]$.

Both of these phase changes are dependent upon the value of z at which the tissue starts. The phase changes induced by gradients for stationary and moving protons are shown diagrammatically in Figures 13-4 and 13-5.

Suppose that at time t = T, the gradient is reversed and is left on from time t = T to time t = 2T (Figure 13-6). For stationary tissue, this will induce a phase change equal to $-\gamma\Delta BzT$. At time t = T, the moving tissue will be located at z coordinate z+VT. Over the interval from t = T to t = 2T, this moving tissue will undergo a phase change of $-[\gamma\Delta B(z+VT)T + (1/2)\gamma V\Delta BT^2]$, where z has been replaced by z+VT. This is equal to $-[\gamma\Delta BzT+(3/2)\gamma V\Delta BT^2]$. Note the negative sign in front of this phase change because the gradient direction has been reversed.

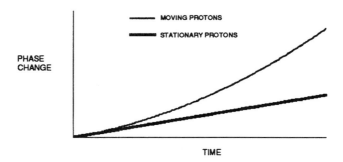

FIGURE 13-4. As a constant gradient is applied, the phase change for moving protons is greater than that for stationary protons.

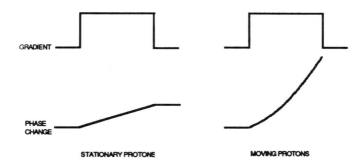

FIGURE 13-5. Same as Figure 13-4 with gradients shown.

Consider the effect of applying both gradients sequentially. Simply add the phase changes calculated for each gradient separately. For stationary tissue, the total phase change is equal to $\gamma\Delta BzT - \gamma\Delta BzT$, which is equal to zero. For tissue moving at constant velocity V, the absolute value of the total phase change is equal to $|(1/2)\gamma V\Delta BT^2 - (3/2)\gamma V\Delta BT^2|$, which is equal to $\gamma V\Delta BT^2$.

Therefore, if sequential gradients of equal magnitude and duration but opposite direction are applied to stationary tissue, no net phase change will occur. On the other hand, if sequential gradients of equal magnitude and duration but opposite direction are applied to tissue moving at constant velocity V (along the direction of the gradient), the net phase change has magnitude $\gamma V\Delta BT^2$. Whether this is a positive or negative absolute phase change is determined by the direction of flow and the direction of the gradients.

Now VT = d is equal to the distance traveled during each gradient application, ΔB is the gradient strength, and T is the time over which each gradient is applied. Therefore, the phase change is directly proportional to the product of distance traveled, gradient strength, and time of application of the gradient. The constant of proportionality is the gyromagnetic ratio γ. Note also that the dependence upon the

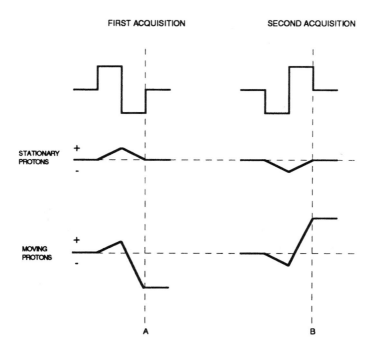

FIGURE 13-6.   In (A), a balanced gradient is applied with a positive first lobe and a negative second lobe. Stationary protons undergo a positive phase change during the first lobe of the gradient and an equal negative phase change during second lobe. The net phase change for stationary protons is zero. Moving protons undergo a positive phase change during the first lobe of the gradient and a much larger negative phase change during second lobe. The moving protons undergo a net negative phase change. In (B), the gradient is reversed so that the first lobe is negative and the second lobe is positive. The stationary protons again undergo no net phase change. The moving protons undergo a net positive phase change [equal in magnitude to the net negative phase change of moving protons in (A)].

starting position (i.e., the starting value of z) has vanished when the sequential gradients are applied.

Suppose such sequential balanced gradients (usually referred to as **flow-encoding** gradients) are added to a GRE sequence along the z direction. Then the measured signal from each voxel will have its phase altered depending upon its velocity of motion along the z direction. If a voxel contains only stationary tissue, then the phase alteration caused by the flow-encoding gradients will be zero. Suppose that a voxel contains intravascular flowing protons with velocity V along the z direction. Then the flow-encoding gradient will induce a phase change of magnitude $\gamma V \Delta B T^2$ for the intravascular protons.

Suppose the same GRE sequence is repeated twice with the direction of the flow-encoding gradients reversed between acquisitions. That is, if for the first acquisition, the flow-encoding gradient is $B(x,y,z) = (B_o + z\Delta B)$ from $t = 0$ to $t = T$, and $B(x,y,z) = -(B_o + z\Delta B)$ from $t = T$ to $t = 2T$. Then, for the second acquisition, the flow-encoding gradient is $B(x,y,z) = -(B_o + z\Delta B)$ from $t = 0$ to $t = T$, and $B(x,y,z) = (B_o + z\Delta B)$ from $t = T$ to $t = 2T$.

The phase change induced by the flow-encoding gradients in stationary tissue is zero for both acquisitions. The phase change induced by the flow-encoding gradients in the moving tissue has the same magnitude for both acquisitions, namely $\gamma V\Delta BT^2$, but has opposite direction (or sign). Therefore, the phase difference between signals from the two acquisitions for the moving tissue has magnitude $2\gamma V\Delta BT^2$.

If the signals from the two acquisitions are subtracted (not the pixel signal intensities but the actual signals, which have a phase difference), the difference signal will be zero for stationary tissue and possibly nonzero for moving tissue (depending on the value of $2\gamma V\Delta BT^2$). Let $\Delta\phi = 2\gamma V\Delta BT^2$. If $\Delta\phi$ equals any multiple of $360°$ (i.e., an integral number of cycles), then the difference signal will be zero for moving tissue as well as stationary tissue. However, if $\Delta\phi$ is not equal to a multiple of $360°$, then the difference signal for the moving tissue will be nonzero. In fact, the difference signal in moving tissue is maximized by having $\Delta\phi = 180°$. When signals that are out of phase by $180°$ are subtracted, this is equivalent to adding the two signals together in phase.

If an image is formed such that the signal intensity in each pixel is equal to the intensity of the difference signal as described above, then stationary tissue will have no signal and moving tissue will have signal whose intensity is dependent upon the velocity along the flow-encoding direction. The contrast in such images is therefore dependent upon the phase change induced by the flow-encoding gradient. This technique is therefore referred to as **PC MRA**.

In order to selectively image vessels with a particular flow velocity V, the flow-encoding gradient strength (ΔB) and/or time of application of the flow-encoding gradient can be adjusted such that $2\gamma V\Delta BT^2 = 180°$. This will maximize the signal in vessels with flow velocity V. However, if the flow velocity in a vessel is an odd integral multiple of V (i.e., 3V, 5V, etc.), then the signal in these vessels will also be maximized. This results from the fact that a phase change of $(2N + 1) \times 180° = N \times 360° + 180°$ is equal to a phase change of $180°$. This means that if blood flow is fast enough, the signal in some vessels with velocities well above V may be maximized. This is equivalent to velocity aliasing along the flow-encoding direction.

Suppose it is desired to selectively image arterial flow with velocity V_A. Then ΔB and T will be chosen such that $2\gamma V_A\Delta BT^2 = 180°$. The velocity of venous flow (V_V) will be such that $V_V \ll V_A$. Therefore, $2\gamma V_V\Delta BT^2$ will be much less than $180°$ so that venous signal will be minimized. In addition, saturation pulses can also be placed on the venous in-flow side to further reduce venous signal.

Suppose it is desired to selectively image venous flow with velocity V_V. Then ΔB and T will be chosen such that $2\gamma V_V\Delta BT^2 = 180°$. For arterial vessels with flow such that $V_A = 3V_V$ or $V_A = 5V_V$, etc., signal will also be maximized. This results from aliasing along the flow-encoding direction. This can be reduced only by using saturation pulses on the arterial in-flow side of the imaging volume.

In order to flow encode in one direction, two separate acquisitions were acquired and the signals subtracted. The same process can be performed along the y and x directions so that all three directions can be flow encoded. Each such flow encoding must be done separately. It would therefore require six separate acquisitions to flow encode in all directions. The flow encoding gradients cannot be applied simultaneously because there would be no way of distinguishing flow in the different directions. However, there is a means of using only four acquisitions (each with a different combination of flow-encoding gradients) to obtain data with flow encoding in all three directions. This is referred to as Hadamard flow encoding (or multiplexed flow encoding).

Due to the requirement of multiple acquisitions for PC MRA, and the fact that it does not rely on TOF effects, the shortest possible TR is usually used for PC MRA sequences. The user usually prescribes a flow-encoding velocity for a PC MRA acquisition based upon the desire to image arterial or venous flow as well as an estimate of the average flow velocities in different vessels.

3   VASCULAR PROJECTION IMAGES

Regardless of the type of vascular imaging sequence performed, individual sections are the standard form in which the data is acquired. Even if a volume acquisition is obtained, phase encoding is performed along the section select direction in order that the volume be divided into individual sections. For display purposes, it is more convenient to represent the same data as a projection.

Consider a single axial section. The voxels in this section make up a two-dimensional array. The location of each voxel is specified by its x and y coordinates. Suppose we look at rows of voxels parallel to the y axis. The voxels in each such row have the same x coordinate. For each such row, determine the maximal signal intensity among all of the voxels in the row. Assign this signal intensity to the coordinate x. This will transform the two-dimensional array of voxels in the xy plane into a line of voxels along the x axis. If the same thing is done for multiple contiguous axial sections (with each section having a different z coordinate), then this will transform the three-dimensional array (in the xyz coordinate system) into a two-dimensional projection in the xz plane. This corresponds to a coronal or anterior–posterior (AP) projection.

Similarly, if we look at rows of voxels parallel to the x axis in each section, this transformation will correspond to a projection in the yz plane. This is a sagittal (or lateral) projection. Likewise, we can look at rows of voxels along any arbitrary direction and form projections. The signal intensity of each voxel in the projection corresponds to the maximum signal intensity in each such row. Since voxels are displayed as pixels in the final image, this technique is referred to as a maximum intensity pixel (MIP) projection. When vascular studies are performed, it is customary to obtain projections in many directions.

This projection method can result in image artifacts. Each pixel in the projection image will have two dimensions: a length and a height. The length of each pixel in the projection will equal the corresponding length of the pixel in the original section. The height of each pixel will equal the thickness of each section. If the sections are relatively thick, the pixels in the projection image will be relatively large and apparent. This can result in the so called venetian blind artifact. The readily apparent pixel size gives the appearance of lines through the image. This effect can be minimized by using very thin sections. This is easily accomplished with a volume acquisition by using a smaller volume or additional phase-encoding steps along the volume direction.

If individual contiguous sections are used, reduction of this artifact is more difficult. Again, thinner sections would reduce the artifact. However, the thinner the sections that are used, the lower the S/N of the image. Since each section is acquired separately, the sections can be made to overlap. For example, suppose 3-mm-thick axial sections are obtained. Each section has a corresponding thickness along the z axis. Suppose two adjacent sections are obtained, with one extending from z = 0 to z = 3 and the other extending from z = 3 to z = 6. These sections do not overlap. On the other hand, suppose two adjacent axial sections are obtained, with one extending from z = 0 to z = 3 and the other extending from z = 1 to z = 4. These sections would have a 2-mm overlap.

By using such an overlap, the projection images will have a smoother appearance with reduced venetian blind artifact. This technique of overlapping sections is usually referred to by the acronym MOTSA, which stands for multiple overlapping thin section angiography.

14 MR Image Artifacts

1   ZIPPER ARTIFACT

When using spin echo pulse sequences, section selective 180° RF pulses are used to create spin echoes. The profile of a pulse is defined as the RF energy of the pulse as a function of position along the section select direction. Ideally, all RF pulses would have a rectangular profile (Figure 14-1A). This means that the RF energy would immediately fall off to zero at the edges of the section to be excited. However, real 180° RF pulses do not have a perfectly rectangular profile. Instead, the energy of real RF pulses will fall off to zero over a small distance outside of the section being excited (Figure 14-1B).

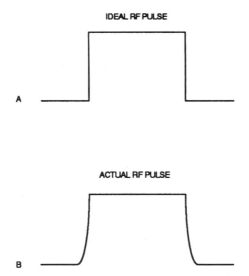

FIGURE 14-1 A & B.   In (A), an ideal RF pulse is shown to have a rectangular profile. An actual RF pulse (B) will not be perfectly rectangular.

Therefore, at the edges of a section, tissue just outside of the section may experience a less than 180° pulse. This will result in the creation of some transverse magnetization within the tissue adjacent to the section actually being excited. This transverse magnetization will emit a signal. However, since the phase-encoding gradients of a conventional spin echo sequence are applied before the 180° pulse, this transverse magnetization will not experience the phase-encoding gradients.

Suppose the center of the FOV is located at the origin of the xyz coordinate system. Suppose the frequency-encoding direction is along the x axis and that the phase-encoding direction is along the y axis. The phase-encoding gradients are symmetric with respect to the axis of the phase-encoding direction. This means that the strength of the phase-encoding gradient at the point (x,y) is proportional to the value of the y coordinate. In this case, the phase-encoding gradient is of equal magnitude but opposite direction at the points (x,y) and (x,−y). Therefore, any source of signal located at points along the x axis (i.e., points with a y coordinate of zero) will undergo a zero increment in phase between phase-encoding gradients.

Likewise, any received signal that undergoes a zero phase increment between phase-encoding steps will be assigned a y coordinate of zero in the displayed image. Tissue excited outside of the section of interest by imperfect 180° pulses will undergo zero phase increment between phase-encoding gradients. All of the signal from this tissue will therefore be displayed along a line passing through the center of the FOV (i.e., along the frequency-encoding axis). Since this line represents signal from a relatively large amount of tissue, it will be of relatively high intensity. This line of signal will be superimposed on the underlying tissue within the image. It often has the appearance of alternating segments of increased and decreased signal, hence the descriptive term **zipper artifact** (Figure 14-2).

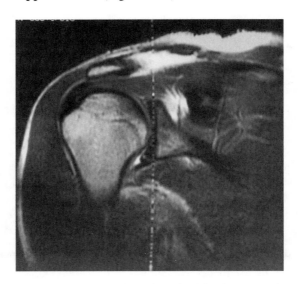

FIGURE 14-2.   Image obtained through the right shoulder shows prominent zipper artifact.

Zipper artifact can be prevented by using more precise RF pulses. It is also prevented by using a trilobed section selective gradient for the 180° pulses. The third lobe of the gradient (sometimes referred to as the crusher lobe) will dephase the signal in tissues that were not excited by the original 90° pulse. This can be seen as follows:

Any tissue that was excited by the original 90° pulse will have transverse magnetization prior to application of the 180° pulse. This transverse magnetization will therefore experience all three lobes of the section selective gradient for the 180° pulse. This is a balanced gradient so that it induces no net phase change in tissue exposed to the entire gradient. However, tissue that has transverse magnetization created by the 180° pulse itself will experience only the second half of the middle lobe and the entire third lobe. This will no longer be balanced and will therefore induce dephasing and signal loss in such tissues. This helps eliminate the signal from tissue outside of the section of interest (Figure 14-3).

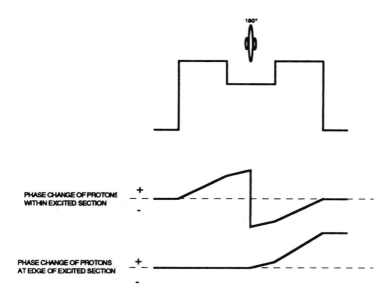

FIGURE 14-3. A trilobed gradient is shown with the first and third lobes being of greater magnitude than the second lobe. All stationary protons within the excited section undergo a positive phase change during the first half of the gradient. This is converted to a negative phase change by the 180° pulse. During the second half of the gradient, the negative phase change is canceled. The net phase change of these protons is therefore zero. Protons outside of the section that are excited by the 180° pulse experience only the second half of the gradient and therefore undergo a net positive phase change while the gradient is on.

There is one other method that is used to help eliminate the signal from the tissue outside of the section of interest. This is referred to as phase cycling (also sometimes referred to as chopper averaging). This technique can be employed only when the NSA is a multiple of 2. Suppose NSA = 2. The phase of the 180° RF pulse can be reversed for the two signal acquisitions. What does this do?

Suppose a 90° RF pulse is applied to a section of tissue. This will create magnetization in the transverse xy plane. The effect of a 180° pulse on transverse magnetization is to rotate it 180°. Suppose the rotation is clockwise around the y axis. Then, for example, if transverse magnetization is oriented along the positive x axis at the time of the 180° pulse, it will be rotated to the negative x axis by the pulse. It does not actually matter whether the rotation is clockwise or counterclockwise. The effect on the transverse magnetization will be the same.

However, suppose the 180° pulse actually acts as a 90° pulse at the edges of a section. Then, the direction of rotation will make a difference. In this tissue, the 180° pulse is acting as a 90° pulse and therefore rotating longitudinal magnetization into the transverse plane. The rotation is still around the y axis. Therefore, if the rotation is counterclockwise, the transverse magnetization will be rotated onto the negative x axis. If the rotation is clockwise, the transverse magnetization will be rotated onto the positive x axis. These two positions are exactly 180° out of phase.

By alternating the direction of rotation of the 180° pulse, the signal from tissue outside of the section of interest will be completely out of phase for the two measurements. There is no effect for tissue within the section of interest. Hence, when the two signals are averaged, the signal from tissue outside of the section of interest will cancel. This is another means of eliminating zipper artifact. Most modern MRI systems employ trilobed section selective 180° pulses as well as phase cycling to eliminate zipper artifact.

2   CENTRAL POINT AND CENTRAL LINE ARTIFACT

This artifact arises from direct current (DC) offsets. The MR signal is actually recorded as an induced voltage in the receiver coil. Ideally, when there is zero signal, there will be zero voltage registered. If there is a defect in the receiver electronics, there may be a small constant voltage registered even in the absence of a signal. This small constant voltage (which has an associated small induced current) is referred to as a direct current offset. It is equivalent to having a constant (i.e., non–time varying) value added to the signal. It can be shown mathematically that the Fourier transform of such a constant signal is a voltage spike at the center frequency of the spectrum.

If the DC offset remains constant, such a voltage spike will have zero phase increment between signal measurements and will have the same center frequency (i.e., 63.87 MHz). It will therefore be displayed as a point of increased signal intensity at the center of the FOV (**central point artifact**). If the DC offset changes in a periodic manner between phase-encoding steps, then it will be displayed along the line of the phase-encoding axis (identical to phase ghosting). This is referred to as a **central line artifact**.

3   RF PENETRATION ARTIFACT

When an excitation pulse is applied to a sample, it is assumed that all portions of the sample experience the same energy of excitation. That is, it is assumed that when, for example, a 90° RF pulse is applied, all portions of the sample experience a 90° pulse. However, as more peripheral portions of a sample absorb RF energy, there will be less RF energy available for the central portions. Therefore, an excitation that produces a 90° pulse in the peripheral portion of a sample may produce only a 75° excitation pulse in the more central portions of the sample (with diminishing degrees of excitation as one goes from peripheral to central portions).

By applying additional RF energy, one can achieve a 90° excitation centrally, but at the price of a greater than 90° excitation peripherally. Either way, the excitation may be heterogeneous throughout a sample. This can lead to artifactual changes in signal intensity that are dependent only on depth within a sample rather than on local values of T1, T2, or proton density. This is referred to as **RF penetration artifact**. This will be worse for larger objects. In general, circularly polarized RF pulses produce more uniform excitation than linearly polarized pulses and will therefore have less RF penetration artifact.

4   DATA CLIPPING ARTIFACT

Using a decimal number system, all numbers are expressed as sums of powers of 10. For example, $123 = (1 \times 10^2) + (2 \times 10^1) + (3 \times 10^0)$, where $10^2 = 100$, $10^1 = 10$, and $10^0 = 1$. This can be denoted as 123_{10}. All computers use a binary number system to store data. Using a binary number system, all numbers are expressed as sums of powers of 2. For example, $123_{10} = (1 \times 2^6) + (1 \times 2^5) + (1 \times 2^4) + (1 \times 2^3) + (0 \times 2^2) + (1 \times 2^1) (1 \times 2^0) = 1111011_2$. Using a binary number system, all values are represented as a series of zeroes and ones. That is, all digits are one of two values. Each binary digit (that is, each zero or one) is referred to as a **bit**. A series of eight bits is referred to as a **byte**.

If, for example, n bits are available for number storage, what is the largest number of data points that can be stored? The answer is 2^n. For example, if two bits are available for storage, then 00, 01, 10, and 11 are the only binary numbers available. If eight bits are available for storage, then $2^8 = 256$ data points can be stored. Regardless of the unit of measurement, a so called "eight bit" ADC can store a range of only 256 different values. The difference between the highest and lowest values (i.e., the range of values) is referred to as the dynamic range of the ADC.

For example, suppose it is known that the highest and lowest voltages induced by the signal (after amplification) are ±4V. Using an eight-bit ADC, we can store voltages in increments $8V/256 = (1/32)V$. In order to accommodate both positive and negative voltages, it is customary to assign a positive voltage to the first 128 binary numbers (i.e., 00000000 to 01111111) and to assign a negative voltage to the last 128 binary numbers (i.e., 10000000 to 11111111). Using this scheme, the first digit of each binary number tells its sign (i.e., a 0 first digit indicates a positive voltage and a 1 first digit indicates a negative voltage).

Should a voltage lie outside of the expected range (say, for example, a voltage of +5V in the example given above), it will be assigned a binary number corresponding to a negative voltage. 5V would be assigned the same binary number as –1V. Likewise, 6V would be assigned the same binary number as –2V. In this manner, if a voltage should exceed the range of values that can be handled by the ADC, it will not be assigned the correct binary number. It will, in essence, undergo aliasing. This is also referred to as **data clipping**.

When an MR signal is measured, it is amplified prior to the actual signal sampling process. The signal is amplified so that the maximal amplified signal does not exceed the capabilities of the ADC. If this is not done, data clipping will occur. Usually, the degree of signal amplification is determined during the prescan process. The receiver amplifier "gain" setting is adjusted appropriately for the ADC. Gain simply means the degree of amplification.

However, on some imaging systems, the prescan process includes an excitation of only the center section of a multisection acquisition. In this case, it can determine the gain setting for the center section only. It is possible that other sections will emit a stronger signal. In order to allow for this, the gain setting is usually chosen to be a percentage (commonly 50%) of the maximal signal from the center section. This usually gives an acceptable margin of error. Using the 50% gain, other sections could have a maximal signal of up to twice that of the center section without getting data clipping.

It should be noted that the portion of the prescan process used to set the receive gain is performed with the lowest strength phase-encoding gradient step (i.e., with no phase-encoding gradient). This phase-encoding gradient will have the highest signal.

5 GEOMETRIC DISTORTION ARTIFACT

Consider two point sources of signal oriented along the frequency-encoding direction separated by a distance D cm. Suppose the signal bandwidth is chosen to be ±16 kHz and suppose the FOV is equal to 32 cm. The strength of the read gradient is adjusted so that the frequency change across the FOV is 32 kHz/32 cm. This corresponds to a frequency change of 1 kHz/cm across the FOV. Therefore, if there were no local distortions of the magnetic field, the two point sources would emit signals with a frequency difference of D kHz. This would be displayed as a separation of D cm in the final image.

Consider a distortion of the local magnetic field near the two point sources. Suppose this distortion results in a frequency difference of only D/2 kHz between the two sources. This would be displayed as a separation of D/2 cm in the final image. That is, the distance between the two sources would be shrunk (by a factor of 2). On the other hand, suppose the distortion results in a frequency difference of 2D kHz between the two sources. This would be displayed as a separation of 2D cm in the final image. That is, the distance between the two sources would be expanded (by a factor of 2).

The same argument applies to the phase-encoding direction. Any local field distortions will alter the expected phase increment. Therefore, distortions of the local magnetic field of any cause (and along either the frequency- or phase-encoding directions) can result in objects being shrunk, expanded, curved, twisted, etc. The distortion of the object is directly related to the distortion of the local magnetic field. Distortions of the local magnetic field would be most commonly caused by magnetic objects or imperfections of the applied gradients.

6 MAGNETIC FIELD PERTURBATION ARTIFACTS

6.1 FIELD INHOMOGENEITY

If the imperfections in the main magnetic field are of a magnitude comparable to the gradients used during the imaging process, then significant image artifacts can result. Geometric distortions that can result have already been discussed. In addition, if there are large regions that have significant field inhomogeneity, this can result in significant signal loss from dephasing. This is usually manifest as a dark (or shaded) area in the image and is usually referred to as "shading." The presence of this artifact usually indicates a problem with the shimming of the main magnetic field.

6.2 ARTIFACT FROM METALLIC OBJECTS

If a metallic object is present within a patient, it may have a different magnetic susceptibility than the surrounding soft tissues. The magnetic susceptibility of an object is a measure of the strength of the magnetic field induced within the object by the applied external magnetic field. Objects with a magnetic susceptibility that is significantly differently from soft tissue will have a significantly different internal magnetic field, compared with soft tissue, even when both are exposed to the same external magnetic field.

This will result in field inhomogeneity in regions close to such objects. This effect is severe for ferromagnetic objects (such as magnetic stainless steel), but may be minimal for nonmagnetic metals. What is the appearance of the artifact caused by such objects? Since metal objects contain no source of MR signal, they should appear as a signal void. However, some unusual appearances can occur at the edges of such objects. The local magnetic field strength in tissue near the edges of a ferromagnetic object will be increased. The increase in field strength will drop off as one moves further from the object.

The frequency-encoding gradient is turned on during the signal measurement process. This gradient induces small changes in the local magnetic field strength as a function of position along the frequency-encoding direction. Therefore, the signal emitted by a given voxel should have a frequency dependent upon the positional coordinate of the voxel along the frequency-encoding direction. The phase-encoding gradient is applied along a direction perpendicular to the read direction. This gradient provides the spatial coordinate of a voxel along the phase-encoding axis.

Suppose the frequency-encoding gradient is along the x axis and that the phase-encoding gradient is along the y axis. An object being imaged consists of a two-dimensional array of voxels. Each voxel has a unique two-dimensional spatial coordinate. A given row of voxels (i.e., a series of voxels parallel to the x axis) will all have the same y coordinate, and a given column of voxels (i.e., a series of voxels parallel to the y axis) will all have the same x coordinate.

Suppose all signal measurements are performed in the absence of the read gradient. This means that all voxels will emit signal of the same frequency. Therefore, only position along the y (or phase-encoding) axis will be discernible. Hence, the image will collapse to a line of pixels along the y axis. The signal in each pixel will equal the sum of the signals from each row of voxels within the object being imaged.

We can now account for the characteristic linear (or sometimes curvilinear) band of markedly increased signal seen at the edge of the signal void from a ferromagnetic object. Recall that tissue located near the edges of a ferromagnetic object will have an increase in the local magnetic field. Suppose the increase in local magnetic field caused by a ferromagnetic object happens to offset the decrease in the local field that would otherwise be caused by the frequency-encoding gradient. Suppose this occurs in portions of multiple rows of consecutive voxels along the frequency direction. Then all such voxels within each row will experience the same field strength while the read gradient is on, and hence they will all emit signal of the same frequency.

Therefore, for each such row (or portion of a row) of voxels, the net signal will collapse to a single pixel in the final image. These single pixels will be oriented in a linear (or curvilinear) column along the phase-encoding direction. This column of pixels will have very high signal intensity because each pixel in the column represents signal from multiple voxels along the frequency direction. Therefore, the appearance of a ferromagnetic object will often be a signal void surrounded by a thin linear or curvilinear band of increased signal intensity on one side (Figure 14-4).

6.3   MAGNETIC SUSCEPTIBILITY EFFECTS

Magnetic susceptibility effects are similar to those described above for metallic objects. Their origin is the same. At the interface of tissues with different magnetic susceptibility, there will be local changes in the magnetic field strength. If these changes are of a magnitude similar to the magnitude of the read gradient, then an area of signal void with an artifactual band of increased signal intensity on one side can be seen at the interface. However, if these changes are of smaller magnitude, then a small area of relative signal void only will be seen.

Small areas of signal void or decreased signal intensity are often seen at the interface of air and soft tissue or bone and soft tissue. Such artifacts are due to relatively small susceptibility changes.

7   CHEMICAL SHIFT ARTIFACT

There are several different types of protons contained within lipids. Some lipid protons are bound to carbon atoms that participate in double or triple bonds with adjacent carbon atoms. These protons are referred to as olefinic protons. However, most lipid protons are bound to carbon atoms that participate in single bonds with adjacent carbon atoms and are referred to as nonolefinic (or methyl) protons.

When exposed to the same external magnetic field strength, water protons and nonolefinic lipid protons will not experience the same magnetic field at the molecular level. This is due to slight differences in molecular structure. On the other hand, water protons and olefinic lipid protons will experience essentially the same magnetic field at the molecular level. However, since most lipid protons are nonolefinic, the term lipid protons in the discussion that follows will refer to nonolefinic lipid protons.

At a field strength of 1.5 T, the resonance frequency of water protons is approximately 220 Hz greater than that of lipid protons. The position of a signal along the frequency-encoding direction is determined by the frequency of the signal. This causes a positional misregistration of voxels containing lipid protons along the frequency-encoding direction, with a positional shift toward the direction of decreasing frequencies.

At a planar lipid–water interface, this positional misregistration can cause two effects. A linear band of pixels with decreased signal intensity occurs at the interface when lipid is on the low-frequency side of the frequency-encoding direction (with

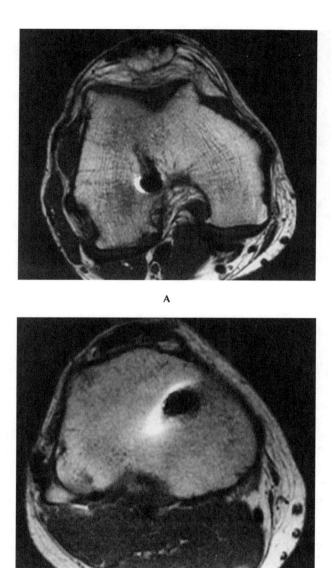

FIGURE 14-4 A&B. (A) Image obtained through the level of the distal femur in a patient with an ACL graft and metal screws. Note the curvilinear increased signal around the region of the femoral screw. Similar artifact is seen in (B) at the level of a tibial screw.

respect to water). This results from the lipid pixels being shifted *away* from the water pixels, which leaves pixels on the lipid side of the interface with absent signal. A linear band of pixels with increased signal intensity occurs at the interface when lipid is on the high-frequency side of the frequency-encoding direction (with respect to water). This results from the lipid pixels being shifted *toward* the water pixels,

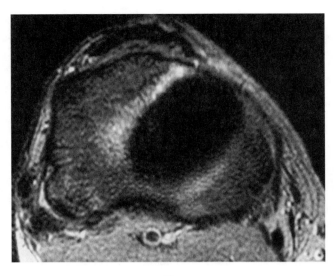

C

FIGURE 14-4 C. GRE image obtained at same level as in (B) shows marked increase in artifact from the metallic screw.

which causes pixels on the water side of the interface to have signal intensity equal to the sum of the lipid- and water-containing pixels (Figure 14-5).

Suppose the signal bandwidth is ±16 kHz along the frequency-encoding direction. If the size of the frequency matrix is 256, then this corresponds to a frequency change of 32,000 Hz/(256 pixels) = 125 Hz per pixel. Therefore, the chemical shift of the position of lipid protons will correspond to a shift of 220 Hz/(125 Hz per pixel) = 220/125 pixels = ~1.76 pixels. This means that the position of voxels containing lipid protons will be shifted by 1 ¾ pixels along the frequency-encoding direction with respect to water protons.

What about chemical shift artifact along the phase-encoding direction? Along the phase-encoding direction, position is determined by the incremental phase change of the signal between phase-encoding steps. The maximal increment in phase occurs at the ends of the FOV. In order to avoid aliasing, this maximal increment in phase must not exceed one-half cycle. Therefore, for a given FOV, the strength of the phase-encoding gradient is always adjusted so as not to exceed a phase increment of more than one-half cycle at the ends of the FOV. The phase increment at more central positions is even less than one-half cycle. The time of application of the phase-encoding gradient is usually kept constant.

The phase-encoding gradient induces phase changes by causing a transient difference in precessional frequency between protons in adjacent voxels. For equal gradient strengths, the absolute phase change of lipid protons will be slightly less than that of water protons at the same location. This results from the slight difference in precessional frequency of water and lipid protons when exposed to the same external field strength. However, the increment in phase between successive phase-encoding steps will be the same for water and lipid protons. This is because the

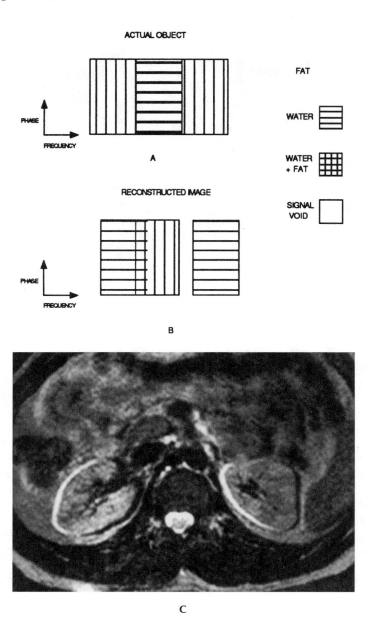

FIGURE 14-5 A, B & C. (A) A water-containing object is surrounded on both sides by fat. In the graphical representation of the reconstructed image (B), the position of fat protons is shifted along the frequency-encoding direction. (C) MR image through the kidneys, which are water-containing structure surrounded by fat. The position of the fat is misregistered along the frequency-encoding direction (left to right). Fat is shifted toward the low frequency side (partient left in the image) since the precessional frequency of fat is less than that of water. Where fat overlaps the water, the signal will be increased relatively. On the opposite side, there is a signal void where there no longer is any fat (or water).

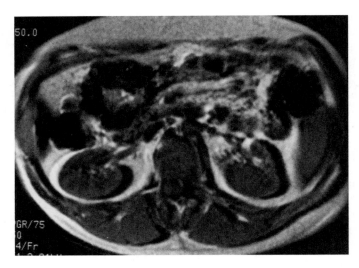

D

FIGURE 14-5 D. Image obtained at similar level as in (C) using a narrow bandwidth (±4 kHz) to exaggerate the chemical shift artifact.

phase increment is dependent only on the increment in gradient strength between phase-encoding steps. This will be the same for all chemical species.

For example, let's examine the phase increment in a water pixel located at the end of the FOV versus the phase increment in a lipid pixel located at the end of the FOV. Assume that the phase-encoding gradient is turned on for 2 ms. Suppose the initial phase-encoding gradient strength induces a frequency change of ±0.25 kHz for water protons at the ends of the FOV. This is equal to 250 c/s, or 0.25 c/ms. Since the phase-encoding gradient is on for 2 ms , this will induce a phase change of ±0.5 cycles for a voxel containing water protons. The difference in precessional frequency between lipid and water protons is 220 Hz = 0.22 c/ms. Therefore, the same gradient will induce a phase change of (0.25 − 0.22) × 2 cycles = 0.06 cycles for a voxel containing lipid protons at the end of the FOV.

The next phase-encoding step will use a gradient strength that induces a frequency change of ±0.5 kHz for water protons at the end of the FOV. This will induce a phase change of ±1.0 cycle (0.5 c/ms × 2 ms = 1.0 cycle). This corresponds to a phase increment of ±(1.0 − 0.5) cycles = ±0.5 cycles from the prior phase-encoding gradient. The same gradient will induce a phase change of (0.5 − 0.22) × 2 cycles = 0.56 cycles for a voxel containing lipid protons at the end of the FOV. This corresponds to a phase increment of ±(0.56 − 0.06) cycles = ±0.5 cycles. Therefore, although the absolute phase change for each phase-encoding gradient is different for water and lipid voxels, the incremental phase change between sequential phase-encoding gradients is the same. Since the incremental phase change between sequential phase-encoding gradients is the same for both water and lipid voxels, there will be no positional misregistration along the phase-encoding direction.

What about the section select direction? In order to selectively excite a section of tissue, a gradient is applied along the section select direction. This causes the resonance frequencies of the protons in the sample to vary as a function of position along the section select direction. Suppose the section select gradient strength is such that the water protons within a certain section of tissue have resonance frequencies in the range 63.87 MHz $\pm$ ΔB Hz. If an excitation pulse contains RF radiation of the same frequency range, then it will selectively excite only protons with corresponding resonance frequencies.

What happens to the lipid protons? The actual region of lipid protons excited will be shifted along the section select direction, causing a misexcitation. The degree of shift, expressed as a percentage of the section thickness, is equal to $\Delta B/220$. The direction of the shift is along the low-frequency side of the section select gradient. This exactly corresponds to positional misregistration along the frequency-encoding direction. Hence, a portion of the lipid within the section to be excited will actually remain unexcited, and a portion of lipid outside of the section to be excited will itself be excited (provided that lipid is present within the tissue on the low-frequency side of the section select gradient).

The lower the bandwidth of the section select gradient, the greater the degree of chemical shift misexcitation that will occur. Therefore, it seems desirable to use as high a bandwidth as possible for the section select gradient. However, the higher the bandwidth of the section select gradient, the greater the gradient strength required. Most high-field-strength MRI systems can achieve a gradient strength of 1.0–1.5 G/cm. Using the higher number of 1.5 G/cm, this corresponds to a frequency change of (63.87 MHz/15,000 G) $\times$ (1.5 G/cm) = 6387 Hz/cm. The minimum section thickness on most systems is 0.2 cm = 2 mm. This corresponds to a frequency change of 6387 Hz/cm $\times$ 0.2 cm = 1276 Hz.

Therefore, most high-field-strength MRI systems will use a bandwidth of 1276 Hz for the section select gradient. The corresponding chemical shift misexcitation along the section select direction will be 220/1276 = ~17%. If, for example, it was desired to obtain a 1.0-mm-thick section, the bandwidth of the section select gradient could be adjusted to 638 Hz. In this case, the degree of chemical shift misexcitation would be approximately 34%. As a comparison, the degree of chemical shift misregistration along the frequency-encoding direction (for a standard bandwidth of $\pm$16 kHz) will be 220/32,000, which is ~0.7%.

8   RF INTERFERENCE ARTIFACT

Suppose there is an external source of RF radiation at a frequency within the range of frequencies of the signal emitted during the MRI process. This signal will be superimposed on the MR signal and will add a constant frequency component. Since this component does not undergo phase-encoding, it will be projected as a line of signal perpendicular to the frequency-encoding axis (i.e., along the direction of the phase-encoding axis). Sources of such RF interference include radio and television transmissions, electric motors, circuits in elevators, cleaning equipment, CT scanners, pumps, typewriters, computer equipment, etc.

9   TRUNCATION (GIBBS) ARTIFACT

As shown in Chapter 7, a square wave can be represented by a sum of sine functions (i.e., a Fourier series) of increasing frequency and decreasing amplitude. The low-frequency sine functions provide a good approximation to the overall shape of the square wave, and the high-frequency sine functions provide the fine detail needed to represent the edges of the square wave. As more and more sine functions are added, the approximation gets closer and closer to the square wave. If an infinite number of sine waves were added together, it could exactly duplicate the square wave.

When a signal is digitized, multiple samples are obtained. These samples can be used to determine the amplitudes of the sine (and cosine) functions in the Fourier series of the signal. The more samples that are obtained, the greater the number of terms of the Fourier series that can be determined. Since only a finite number of samples can be obtained, the amplitude of only a finite number of sine (and cosine) functions of the Fourier series can be determined.

Gibbs artifact arises when there is a sharp interface between an area of relatively high signal and an area of relatively low signal. When constructing an MR image, if a voxel of high signal intensity is surrounded by low signal intensity voxels, then the signal intensity as a function of position would approximate a square wave.

The MRI process obtains only a finite number of samples along both the frequency-encoding and phase-encoding directions. This is equivalent to using only a finite number of cosine functions (Figure 14-6) to approximate the square wave function. Therefore, the Fourier transform process can only approximate a square wave function. In fact, it can be shown mathematically that the approximation to the square wave function using a finite number of sine and cosine functions will have small ripples at the edges (Figure 14-7). These ripples are reconstructed in the final MR image and appear as lines through the image (Figure 14-8).

The spacing between the ripples (and hence the spacing between the lines) is proportional to the number of sine and cosine functions used in the approximation. This, in turn, is equal to the size of the image matrix. In general, these lines are not detectable if the size of the image matrix is 256 or greater. Therefore, Gibbs artifact is virtually never seen along the frequency-encoding direction. In order to reduce Gibbs artifact along the phase-encoding direction, a matrix of 192 or 256 can be used. Gibbs artifact is also commonly referred to as truncation artifact. The term **truncation artifact** is derived from the fact that the data sampling process is ended, or truncated, after a finite number of samples are obtained.

It is a mathematical peculiarity (referred to as the Gibbs phenomenon, named after the physicist Josiah Willard Gibbs) that the amplitude of the ripples does not change with a change in matrix size (i.e., a change in the number of samples). It should be noted that the amplitude of the ripples progressively decreases as one moves away from the edges of the square wave. The effect of using a higher image matrix is to cause the ripples to be more closely spaced, making them less conspicuous through the image.

In neuroradiology MR applications, the Gibbs phenomenon is most troublesome when performing brain imaging. If the phase matrix size is less than 192, curvilinear

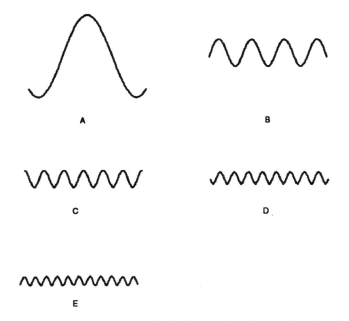

FIGURE 14-6. As one goes from A to E, the frequencies of the cosine functions increase as the amplitudes decrease.

lines corresponding to the shape of the skull–air interface are superimposed across the image. In musculoskeletal imaging, the Gibbs phenomenon is most troublesome when evaluating the menisci of the knee. In this case, Gibbs artifact can arise at the bone–meniscus or cartilage–meniscus interface. This can result in curvilinear lines corresponding to the shape of this interface superimposed on the low-signal menisci.

10 FAST SPIN ECHO–RELATED ARTIFACTS

All of the artifacts seen with conventional spin echo sequences are also seen with FSE sequences. However, there are a number of imaging artifacts that are unique to the FSE sequence. Before discussing these artifacts, we will discuss some basic principles necessary for their understanding.

Consider an MR image of a point source of signal. A point source is a very small source of signal, on the order of a voxel or less in dimension. Suppose the source is located at the origin of the xyz coordinate system. Under ideal conditions, if signal intensity is plotted as a function of position, it will appear as a spike located at the origin. However, the actual plot will appear as a function with a sharp peak located at the origin that falls off to zero on either side of the origin (Figure 14-9). The more accurate the image, the sharper the peak (i.e., the more quickly the signal falls off to zero). Such a function is referred to as the point spread function (PSF). It represents the "spreading" of the image of a point source of signal.

A point source is an artificial construct, because even an individual voxel has a finite dimension. Real objects can, however, be thought of as consisting of multiple

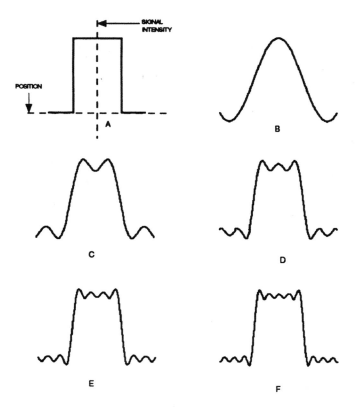

FIGURE 14-7. (A) Representation of a sharp change in signal intensity within an object. For example, this might be seen at the interface of air with subcutaneous fat (when imaging the head or body) or at the interface of meniscus with bone (when imaging the knee). (B) Same as Figure 14-6A. (C) through (F) shows sums of cosine functions of progressively higher frequency and lower amplitude (like those shown in Figure 14-6). The approximation to (A) gets progressively better, but the small ripples at the edges persist. The ripples get more closely spaced, but do not vanish in amplitude.

distinct small regions of homogeneous tissue with identical values of proton density, T1, and T2. An image voxel would approximate such a region. Suppose an axial section (i.e., a section of tissue in the xy plane) of an object being imaged consists of M such regions. The total MR signal is therefore the sum of the individual signals from each of these regions.

Let the function $f_n(x,y)$ be the *true* representation of the image of the n-th region, $1 \leq n \leq M$. Let $g_n(x,y)$ be the actual image of the n-th region. It can be shown mathematically that $g_n(x,y) = p_n(x,y)*f_n(x,y)$, where * denotes an operation referred to as convolution and $p_n(x,y)$ is a PSF. The precise definition of the convolution operation is not important. It suffices to know that the convolution of two functions is a type of multiplication of the two functions. In essence, the above equation states that the convolution of the PSF with the true image gives the actual image. In this

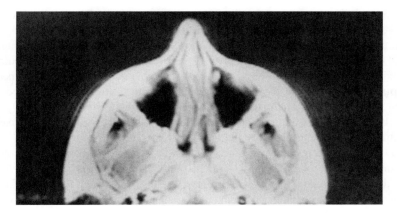

FIGURE 14-8.   Axial image obtained through the level of the midface. The phase direction is from right to left and the phase matrix is 128. Prominent Gibbs artifact is manifest as lines at the edge of the face.

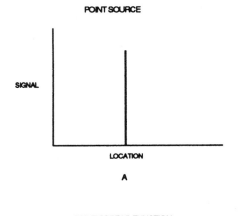

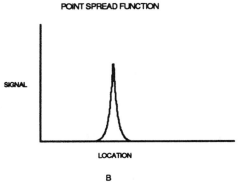

FIGURE 14-9.   (A) The signal from a point source would be a sharp spike. (B) The actual signal is spread along the axis of location.

sense, the PSF is a measure of the distortion of the true image. The sharper the PSF, the more closely the actual image resembles the true image.

Another way of looking at this is as follows. Suppose a single voxel (V_1) emits a signal of amplitude S. Ideally, the pixel (P_1) corresponding to this voxel would be assigned signal of amplitude S, and no signal from this voxel would be assigned to other pixels. However, the location of this signal in the actual image may be distributed over more than one pixel, and the amplitude of the signal in pixel P_1 may be less than S. The distribution and amplitude of the signal from a certain voxel in the actual image is determined by the PSF for that voxel.

Now let us return to the equation $g_n(x,y) = p_n(x,y)*f_n(x,y)$. Recall that the object being imaged was broken up into M small regions, each region having the same proton density, T1, and T2 values. Therefore, the PSF must be a function of these variables. In fact, for conventional spin echo sequences, it can be shown that $p_n(x,y)$ is proportional to $N(H)(1 - e^{-TR/T1})e^{-TE/T2}$, where $N(H)$ is the proton density. Note that with conventional spin echo sequences, the echo time is the same for each phase-encoding step. However, for FSE sequences, the echo time at which each phase-encoded sample is acquired will vary. In the case of FSE sequences, TE becomes a function of the phase-encoding step.

This dependence of TE on the phase-encoding step alters the PSF. It can be shown mathematically that the following effects will occur:

First, if an FSE sequence is used to generate proton density– or T1-weighted images, the PSF will be widened and its amplitude will be diminished. Widening of the PSF corresponds to a blurring effect. Decreased amplitude of the PSF corresponds to a decrease in signal intensity. The shorter the T2 of a particular tissue, the more pronounced these effects will be. Therefore, these effects will be most pronounced for small objects with a short T2 (in this sense, small means on the order of a voxel or less in size).

A qualitative explanation of this effect has already been given in Chapter 10. When an FSE sequence is used to generate proton density– or T1-weighted images, the weak phase-encoding gradients are applied to the early echoes (i.e., those echoes acquired with short TE) and the strong phase-encoding gradients are applied to the late echoes (i.e., those echoes acquired with long TE). The strong phase-encoding gradients cause greater signal loss due to dephasing. Therefore, the combination of a strong phase-encoding gradient and a late echo results in very little signal. However, the signals acquired with the strong phase-encoding gradients provide spatial resolution. If not enough signal is available for these echoes, spatial resolution is lost. This is equivalent to image blurring. This effect will be worse for tissues with a short T2, since the shorter the T2 the less the signal intensity at any given echo time. For a given T2 value, it will also be worse for small objects, which have intrinsically less signal.

Echoes acquired with the weak phase-encoding gradients provide most of the signal in the image. The shorter the T2 of a tissue, the lower the signal intensity at any given echo time (including the early echoes). Tissues with a short T2 will have less signal even for relatively early echoes. Therefore, signal loss will be more pronounced for tissues with a short T2. Again, this effect will be most pronounced for small objects.

As the echo train length is increased, echoes will be acquired at later and later times. This will result in more signal loss for such echoes. An identical effect occurs when a longer echo spacing is used. Therefore, use of a longer echo train length and/or a longer echo spacing will increase image blurring and decrease signal intensity, especially for small objects with a short T2.

Second, if an FSE sequence is used to generate T2-weighted images, the PSF will be narrowed and its amplitude will be increased. Narrowing of the PSF corresponds to a sharpening of the image. This is most pronounced at the interface of two areas of tissue with different T2 values, giving an edge enhancement effect, meaning a sharper appearance of the interface. Increased amplitude of the PSF corresponds to an increase in signal intensity. This increase in signal intensity is most pronounced for objects with a long T2 value.

A qualitative explanation of this effect is as follows: When an FSE sequence is used to generate T2-weighted images, the strong phase-encoding gradients are applied to the early echoes (i.e., those echoes acquired with short TE) and the weak phase-encoding gradients are applied to the late echoes (i.e., those echoes acquired with long TE).

The combination of a strong phase-encoding gradient and an early echo results in maximal signal for those echoes acquired with the strong phase-encoding gradients. The signals acquired with the strong phase-encoding gradients provide spatial resolution. The higher signal for these early echoes results in optimal spatial resolution. This is equivalent to a sharper appearing image. This effect will be most apparent at interfaces between tissues with different T2 values. It will also result in a sharper appearance to small objects.

The echoes acquired with the weak phase-encoding gradients provide most of the signal in the image. Using conventional spin echo sequences, T2-weighted images would acquire all echoes, including those with the weak phase-encoding gradients, at a relatively late echo time. Therefore, tissues with a short T2 would have relatively low signal intensity at the time of all echoes. However, with FSE T2-weighted images, the weak phase-encoding gradients will be acquired at late echoes. Tissues with short T2 values may still have substantial signal at this time since weaker phase-encoding gradients are used. This will give a relatively higher signal intensity even to objects with a short T2. Again, this effect will be more pronounced for small objects.

Third, with conventional spin echo sequences, there is no T2 signal decay between different phase-encoding steps, since all echoes are acquired at the same echo time. However, with FSE sequences, there is T2 signal decay between adjacent phase-encoding steps during each TR interval. This signal decay between phase-encoding steps is equivalent to collecting data in a discontinuous manner. Such discontinuities in data collection will result in image artifacts. These artifacts appear as additional signal components along the phase-encoding direction. Thus, their appearance is very similar to phase ghosts. This artifact can be reduced by collecting the data such that T2 decay between adjacent phase-encoding steps is minimized. This is achieved by using the shortest possible echo spacing.

Suggested Readings

CHAPTER 1

Evans, R. D. *The Atomic Nucleus.* New York: McGraw-Hill , 1955.

CHAPTER 2

Schenk, J. F. "The role of magnetic susceptibility in magnetic resonsAnce imaging: MRI magnetic compatibility of the first and second kinds." *Med. Phys.* 1996; 33:815.
Thomas, S. R. and Dixon, R. L., eds. *NMR in Medicine The Instrumentation and Clinical Applications.* New York: American Institute of Physics, 1986.

CHAPTER 3

Purcell, E. M. *Electricity and Magnetism.* New York: McGraw-Hill, 1985.
Thomas, S. R. and Dixon, R. L., eds. *NMR in Medicine The Instrumentation and Clinical Applications.* New York: American Institute of Physics, 1986.

CHAPTER 4

James T. L. and Margulis, A. R., eds. *Biomedical Magnetic Resonance.* San Francisco: Radiology Research and Education Foundation, 1984.
Thomas, S. R. and Dixon, R. L., eds. *NMR in Medicine The Instrumentation and Clinical Applications.* New York: American Institute of Physics, 1986.

CHAPTER 5

Chen C-N. and Hoult, D. I. *Biomedical Magnetic Resonance Technology.* New York: Adam Hilger, 1989.
Homans, S. W. *A Dictionary of Concepts in NMR.* Oxford: Clarendon Press, 1992.
James T. L. and Margulis, A. R., eds. *Biomedical Magnetic Resonance.* San Francisco: Radiology Research and Education Foundation, 1984.
Thomas, S. R. and Dixon, R. L., eds. *NMR in Medicine The Instrumentation and Clinical Applications.* New York: American Institute of Physics, 1986.

CHAPTER 6

Chen C-N. and Hoult, D. I. *Biomedical Magnetic Resonance Technology.* New York: Adam Hilger, 1989.
Homans, S. W. *A Dictionary of Concepts in NMR.* Oxford: Clarendon Press, 1992.

James T. L. and Margulis, A. R., eds. *Biomedical Magnetic Resonance.* San Francisco: Radiology Research and Education Foundation, 1984.

Thomas, S. R. and Dixon, R. L., eds. *NMR in Medicine The Instrumentation and Clinical Applications.* New York: American Institute of Physics, 1986.

CHAPTER 7

Chen C-N. and Hoult, D. I. *Biomedical Magnetic Resonance Technology.* New York: Adam Hilger, 1989.

James T. L. and Margulis, A. R., eds. *Biomedical Magnetic Resonance.* San Francisco: Radiology Research and Education Foundation, 1984.

Thomas, S. R. and Dixon, R. L., eds. *NMR in Medicine The Instrumentation and Clinical Applications.* New York: American Institute of Physics, Inc., 1986.

CHAPTER 8

Chen C-N. and Hoult, D. I. *Biomedical Magnetic Resonance Technology.* New York: Adam Hilger, 1989.

James T. L. and Margulis, A. R., eds. *Biomedical Magnetic Resonance.* San Francisco: Radiology Research and Education Foundation, 1984.

Thomas, S. R. and Dixon, R. L., eds. *NMR in Medicine The Instrumentation and Clinical Applications.* New York: American Institute of Physics, 1986.

CHAPTER 9

Edelstein, W. A., Glover, G. H., Hardy, C. J., and Redington, R. W. "The intrinsic signal-to-noise ratio in NMR imaging." *Magn. Reson. Med.* 1986; 3:605.

Hart, H. R., Jr., Bottomley, P. A., Edelstein, W. A., Karr, S. G., Leue, W. M., Mueller, O., Redington, R. W., Schenck, J. F., Smith, L. S., and Vatis, D. "Nuclear magnetic resonance imaging: Contrast-to-noise ratio as a function of strength of magnetic field." *AJR* 1983; 141:1195.

Johnson, J. B. "Thermal agitation of electricity in conductors." *Phys. Rev.* 1928; 32:97.

Mugler, J. P. and Brookman, J. R. "The optimum data sampling period for maximum signal-to-noise ratio in MR imaging." *Rev. Magn. Reson. Med.* 1988; 3(1):1.

Nyquist, H. "Thermal agitation of electric charge in conductors." *Phys. Rev.* 1928; 32:110.

CHAPTER 10

Bailes, D. R., Gilderdale, D. J., Bydder, G. M., Collins, A. G., and Firmin, D. N. "Respiratory ordered phase encoding (ROPE): A method for reducing respiratory motion artifacts in MR imaging." *JCAT* 1985; 9(4):835.

Dixon, W. T. "Simple proton spectroscopic imaging." *Radiology* 1984; 153:189.

Ehman, R. L., McNamara, M. T., Pallack, M., Hricak, H., and Higgins, C. B. "Magnetic resonance imaging with respiratory gating: Techniques and advantages." *ARRS* 1984; 84:1175.

Enzmann, D. R., Rubin, J. B., DeLaPaz, R., and Wright, A. "Cerebrospinal fluid pulsation: Benefits and pitfalls in MR imaging." *Radiology* 1986;161:773.

Glover, G. H. "Multipoint dixon technique for water and fat proton and susceptibility imaging." *JMRI* 1991; 1:521.

Glover, G. H. and Schneider, E. "Three-point dixon technique for true water/fat decomposition with B_0 inhomogeneity correction." *Magn. Reson. Med.* 1991; 18:371.

Hinks, R. S. and Constable, R. D. "Gradient moment nulling in fast spin echo." *MRM* 1994; 32:698.

Pusey, E., Lufkin, R. B., Brown, R. K. J., Solomon, M. A., Stark, D. D., Tarr, R. W., and Hanafee, W. N. "Magnetic resonance imaging artifacts: Mechanism and clinical significance." *Radiographics* 1986; 6:891.

Pykett, I. L. and Rosen, B. R. "Nuclear magnetic resonance: *In vivo* proton chemical shift imaging. Work in progress." *Radiology* 1983; 149:197.

Runge, V. M., Clanton, J. A., Partain, C. L., and James, A. E. "Respiratory gating in magnetic resonance imaging at 0.5 Tesla." *Radiology* 1984; 151:521.

Szumowsky, J. and Plewes, D. B. "Separation of lipid and water MR imaging signals by chopper averaging in the time domain." *Radiology* 1987; 165:247.

Williams, S. C. R., Horsfield, M. A., and Hall, L. D. "True water and fat MR imaging with use of multiple-echo acquisition." *Radiology* 1989; 173:249.

Wood, M. L. and Henkelman, R. M. "The magnetic field dependence of the breathing artifact." *MRI* 1986; 4:387.

Wood, M. L. and Henkelman, R. M. "Suppression of respiratory motion artifacts in magnetic resonance imaging." *Med. Phys.* 1986; 13(6):794.

CHAPTER 11

GRADIENT ECHO

Bruder, H., Fischer, H., Graumann, R., and Deimling, M. "A new steady-state imaging sequence for simultaneous acquisition of two MR images with clearly different contrasts." *Magn. Reson. Med.* 1988; 7:35.

Chien, D. and Edelman, R. R. "Ultrafast imaging using gradient echoes." *Magn. Reson. Q.* 1991; 7(1):31.

Elster, A. D. "Gradient echo MR imaging: Techniques and acronyms." *Radiology* 1993; 186:1.

Gyngell, M. L. "The steady-state signals in short-repetition-time sequences." *J. Magn. Reson.* 1989; 81:474.

Haacke, E. M., Wielopolski, P. A., and Tkach, J. A. "A comprehensive technical review of short TR, fast, magnetic resonance imaging." *Rev. Magn. Reson. Med.* 1988; 3(2)53.

Haacke, E. M. and Tkach, J. A. "Fast MR imaging: Techniques and clinical applications." *AJR* 1990; 155:951.

Hawkes, R. C. and Patz, S. "Rapid fourier imaging using steady-state free precession." *Magn. Reson. Med.* 1987; 4:9.

Lee, S.Y. and Cho, Z. H. Fast "SSFP gradient echo sequence for simultaneous acquisitions of FID and echo signals." *Magn. Reson. Med.* 1988; 8:142.

Sattin, W., Mareci T. H., and Scott, K. N. "Exploiting the stimulated echo in nuclear magnetic resonance imaging. I. Method." *J. Magn. Reson.* 1985; 64:177.

Wehrli, F. W. "Fast-scan magnetic resonance: Principles and applications." *Magn. Reson. Q.* 1990; 6(3):165.

Wood, M. L., Silver, M., and Runge, V. M. "Optimization of spoiler gradients in flash MRI." *MRI* 1987; 5:455-463.

Fast Spin Echo

Constable, R. T., Anderson, A. W,. Zhong, J., and Gore, J. C. "Factors influencing contrast in fast spin-echo MR imaging." *Magn. Reson. Imag.* 1992; 10:497.

Constable, R. T. and Gore, J. C. "The loss of small objects in variable TE imaging: Implications for FSE, RARE, and EPI." *Magn. Reson. Med.* 1992; 18:9.

Constable, R. T., Smith, R. C., and Gore, J. C. "Coupled-spin fast spin-echo MR imaging." *JMRI* 1993; 3:547.

Hennig, J., Nauerth, A., and Friedburg, H. "RARE imaging: A fast imaging method for clinical MR." *Magn. Reson. Med.* 1986; 3:823.

Melki. P. S., Mulkern, R. V., Panych, L. P., and Jolesz, F. A. "Comparing the FAISE method with conventional dual-echo sequences." *JMRI* 1991; 1:319.

Mulkern, R. V., Melki, P. S., Higuchi, N., and Jolesz, F. A. "Phase-encode order and its effect on contrast and artifact in single-shot RARE sequences." *Med. Phys.* 1991; 18(5):1032.

Mulkern, R. V., Wong, S. T. S., Winalski, C., and Jolesz, F. A. "Contrast manipulation and artifact assessment of 2D and 3D RARE sequences." *Magn. Reson. Imag.* 1990; 8:557.

CHAPTER 12

Axel, L. "Surface coil magnetic resonance imaging." *JCAT* 1984; 8(3):381.

Bydder, G. M., Curati, W. L., Gadian, D. G., Hall, A. S., Harman, R. R., Butsen, P. R., Gilderdale, D. J., and Young, I. R. "Use of closely coupled receiver coils in MR imaging: Practical aspects." *JCAT* 1985; 9(5):987.

Hayes, C. E., Hattes, N., and Roemer, P. B. "Volume imaging with MR phased arrays." *Magn. Reson. Med.* 1991; 18:309.

Hayes, C. E. and Roemer, P. B. "Noise correlations in data simultaneously acquired from multiple surface coil arrays." *Magn. Reson. Med.* 1990; 16:181.

Roemer, P. B., Edelstein, W. A., Hayes, C. E., Souza, S. P., and Mueller, O. M. "The NMR phased array." *Magn. Reson. Med.* 1990; 16:192.

Smith, R. C., Reinhold, C., McCauley, T., Lange, R. C., Constable, R. T., Kier, R., and McCarthy, S. M. "Multicoil high resolution fast spin echo MR Imaging of the female pelvis." *Radiology* 1992; 184:671-675.

CHAPTER 13

Bradley, W. G. and Waluch, V. "Blood flow: Magnetic resonance imaging." *Radiology* 1985; 154:443.

Laub, G. A. and Kaiser, W. A. "MR angiography with gradient motion refocusing." *JCAT* 1988; 12(3):377.

Nishimura, D. G., Jackson, J. I., and Pauly, J. M. "On the nature and reduction of the displacement artifact in flow images. "*Magn. Reson. Med.* 1991; 22:481.

Pelc, N. J., Herfkens, R. J., Shimakawa, A., and Enzmann, D. R. "Phase contrast cine magnetic resonance imaging." *Magn. Reson. Q.* 1991; 7(4):229.

Urchuk, S. T. and Plewes, D. B. "Mechanisms of flow-induced signal loss in MR angiography." *JMRI* 1991; 2:453.

Wang, S. J., Hu, B. S., Macovski, A., and Nishimura, D. G. "Coronary angiography using fast selective inversion recovery." *Magn. Reson. Med.* 1991; 18:417.

CHAPTER 14

Bellon, E. M., Haacke, E. M., Coleman, P. E., Sacco, D. C., Steiger, D. A., and Gangarosa, R. E. *AJR* 1986; 147:1271.

Henkelman, R. M. and Bronskill, M. J." Artifacts in magnetic resonance imaging." *Rev. Magn. Reson. Med.* 1987; 2(2):1.

Laakman, R. W., Kaufman, B., Han, J. S., Nelson, A. D., Clampitt, M., O'Block, A. M., Haaga, J. R., and Alfidi, R. J. "MR imaging in patients with metallic implants." *Radiology* 1985; 157:711.

Low, R. N., Hinks, R. S., Alzate, G. D., and Shimakawa, A. "Fast spin-echo MR imaging of the abdomen: Contrast optimization and artifact reduction." *JMRI* 1994; 4:637.

New, P. F. J., Rosen, B. R., Brady, T. J., Buonanno, R. S., Kistler, J. P., Burt, C. T., Hinshaw, W. S., Newhouse, J. H., Pohost, G. M., and Taveras, J. M. "Potential hazards and artifacts of ferromagnetic and nonferromagnetic surgical and dental materials and devices in nuclear magnetic resonance imaging." *Radiology* 1983; 147:139.

Index